Schema Therapy Exercises and Worksheets

100+ Evidence-Based Techniques for Trauma Recovery, Pattern Breaking, and Emotional Resilience for Therapists, Counselors, and Individual Healing

Vionnet Vilina McKinney

Table of Contents

Introduction

Schema Therapy represents one of the most powerful advances in modern psychotherapy—a treatment approach that addresses the deepest roots of psychological suffering. Unlike traditional therapies that focus primarily on symptoms, Schema Therapy targets the fundamental patterns of thinking, feeling, and behaving that shape our entire experience of life. These patterns, called schemas, form during our earliest years and continue to influence us throughout adulthood, often in ways we don't fully understand.

The beauty of Schema Therapy lies in its recognition that lasting change requires more than just cognitive insight or behavioral modification. It requires healing at the emotional level—touching the wounded parts of ourselves that developed during childhood and continue to cry out for attention, validation, and care. This approach acknowledges that our early experiences don't just influence us; they become part of the very fabric of who we are.

Schema Therapy: Core Concepts and Principles

Schema Therapy emerged from the brilliant mind of Jeffrey Young, who recognized that traditional cognitive-behavioral therapy, while effective for many conditions, fell short when treating individuals with deeply entrenched patterns of dysfunction[1]. Working with clients who seemed resistant to conventional approaches, Young discovered that their difficulties stemmed from much deeper sources—from the fundamental beliefs and emotional patterns established during their formative years.

The foundation of Schema Therapy rests on four core concepts that work together to create a complete understanding of human psychological functioning. **Early Maladaptive Schemas** represent the first cornerstone—these are broad, pervasive themes or patterns that comprise memories, emotions, cognitions, and bodily sensations regarding oneself and one's relationships with others[2]. These schemas develop during childhood or adolescence and are elaborated throughout one's lifetime, often creating self-defeating patterns that persist despite their obvious harm.

Consider the case of **Maria**, a 35-year-old marketing executive who came to therapy complaining of chronic relationship difficulties. Despite her professional success, Maria found herself repeatedly attracted to emotionally unavailable partners who would eventually abandon her. Through Schema Therapy assessment, we identified her core Abandonment schema—a deep belief that people she cares about will inevitably leave her. This schema developed during her childhood when her father left the family without warning when she was eight years old, and her mother became emotionally distant, struggling with depression.

Maria's Abandonment schema didn't just influence her choice of partners; it shaped her entire approach to relationships. She would become intensely clingy early in relationships, desperately seeking reassurance, which ironically pushed partners away and confirmed her worst fears. This pattern had repeated itself countless times, each failed relationship strengthening her belief that she was fundamentally unlovable and destined to be alone.

The second core concept involves **Coping Styles**—the characteristic ways individuals respond to their schemas[3]. Young identified three primary coping styles: surrender, avoidance, and overcompensation. In Maria's case, she alternated between surrender (accepting that she would be abandoned and becoming passive in relationships) and overcompensation (becoming controlling and demanding to prevent abandonment). Neither approach served her well, but these were the only strategies she knew.

Schema Modes represent the third fundamental concept—these are the emotional states and coping responses that are active at any given moment[4]. Unlike schemas, which are relatively stable traits, modes are temporary states that can shift throughout the day. Maria would flip between her Vulnerable Child mode (feeling small, frightened, and desperate for love) and her Demanding Parent mode (becoming critical and controlling when she felt threatened).

2

The fourth concept centers on **Core Emotional Needs**—the universal human requirements that, when unmet during childhood, lead to schema development[5]. These include needs for safety, stability, nurturance, acceptance, autonomy, competence, identity, expression, spontaneity, and realistic limits. Maria's childhood experiences left her with profound unmet needs for stability and nurturance, which continued to drive her adult relationships.

Another compelling example involves **David**, a 42-year-old engineer who struggled with perfectionism and workaholism. David's Unrelenting Standards schema developed in response to parents who provided love and approval only when he achieved at the highest levels. His childhood was filled with academic and athletic achievements, but also with constant pressure and criticism for any perceived shortcoming.

As an adult, David worked 80-hour weeks, never feeling satisfied with his accomplishments. His relationships suffered because he applied the same impossible standards to his wife and children. His Demanding Parent mode drove him relentlessly, while his Vulnerable Child mode felt anxious and inadequate beneath the surface. The cost of maintaining this schema was enormous—chronic stress, strained relationships, and a persistent sense that nothing he did was ever good enough.

The case of **Jennifer**, a 28-year-old teacher, illustrates how multiple schemas can interact to create complex psychological difficulties. Jennifer presented with social anxiety and depression, struggling to maintain friendships and romantic relationships. Assessment revealed three primary schemas: Defectiveness (believing she was fundamentally flawed and unworthy of love), Social Isolation (feeling different from and disconnected from others), and Emotional Deprivation (expecting that her emotional needs would never be met).

These schemas developed in response to childhood bullying and parents who were emotionally cold and critical. Jennifer's coping style involved significant avoidance—she isolated herself to prevent others from discovering her perceived flaws. When forced into social situations, she would retreat into her Detached Protector mode,

3

appearing aloof and disinterested, which prevented genuine connection and reinforced her schemas.

Schema Therapy's approach to healing these deep patterns involves what Young calls **Limited Reparenting**—the therapist provides some of the nurturing, validation, and guidance that the client missed during childhood[6]. This doesn't mean the therapist becomes a parent, but rather that they offer genuine care and concern while maintaining appropriate boundaries. The therapeutic relationship becomes a laboratory for experiencing healthier patterns of connection.

The therapy also employs **Empathic Confrontation**—a delicate balance of understanding and challenge[7]. The therapist validates the client's schemas and coping responses as understandable adaptations to difficult circumstances, while simultaneously helping them recognize how these patterns now create problems in their adult life. This approach avoids the shame and defensiveness that often arise when people feel criticized for their coping mechanisms.

Schema Therapy integrates cognitive, emotional, and behavioral techniques within a unified framework. **Cognitive techniques** help clients identify and challenge schema-driven thoughts and beliefs. **Experiential techniques** such as imagery rescripting and chair work allow clients to process and heal emotional wounds at the feeling level. **Behavioral techniques** help clients break old patterns and establish new, healthier ways of responding to life's challenges.

The **18 Early Maladaptive Schemas** are organized into five domains based on the core needs they represent[8]. The Disconnection and Rejection domain includes schemas like Abandonment, Mistrust/Abuse, Emotional Deprivation, Defectiveness, and Social Isolation. The Impaired Autonomy and Performance domain encompasses Dependence, Vulnerability to Harm, Enmeshment, and Failure schemas. Other-Directedness includes Subjugation, Self-Sacrifice, and Approval-Seeking schemas. The Overvigilance and Inhibition domain contains Negativity, Emotional Inhibition, Unrelenting Standards, and Punitiveness schemas. Finally, Impaired Limits includes Entitlement and Insufficient Self-Control schemas.

Guidelines for Therapists and Self-Help Users

This collection serves dual purposes—providing professional therapists with evidence-based tools while offering individuals the opportunity to work on their own healing. The exercises are designed to be flexible, allowing adaptation to different settings and needs.

For Therapists: Each exercise includes detailed instructions, theoretical background, and guidance for implementation. The tools progress from basic assessment to advanced interventions, allowing you to match techniques to your client's readiness and therapeutic phase. Early exercises focus on education and awareness, while later tools address deeper emotional processing and behavioral change.

Begin with assessment tools to establish a clear understanding of your client's schema profile. Use the Schema Interview Protocol and Young Schema Questionnaire to identify primary schemas and their severity. This foundation guides treatment planning and helps predict potential challenges.

The progression through exercises should match your client's developmental capacity and emotional stability. Clients with significant trauma histories or poor emotional regulation may need extensive preparation before engaging in imagery work or chair techniques. Always prioritize safety and stability over speed of progress.

For Self-Help Users: This collection can support personal growth and healing, but self-awareness and honesty are essential. Start with the assessment tools to understand your own patterns, then work systematically through the exercises that resonate most strongly with your experience.

Maintain realistic expectations about the pace of change. Schema-level healing occurs gradually, often requiring months or years of consistent work. Celebrate small victories and be patient with setbacks, which are normal parts of the healing process.

Consider working with a trained Schema Therapist alongside using these tools. While self-help can be powerful, the support and guidance of a skilled professional can accelerate healing and provide safety during difficult emotional work.

Safety Protocols: Some exercises may trigger intense emotions or memories. If you experience overwhelming distress, suicidal thoughts, or dissociation, stop the exercise and seek professional support immediately. These reactions aren't failures—they're signs that your emotional system needs additional care and support.

Safety Considerations and Contraindications

Schema Therapy work can activate powerful emotions and memories, making safety considerations paramount. Understanding contraindications and risk factors helps ensure that healing work proceeds safely and effectively.

Absolute Contraindications include active psychosis, severe dissociative disorders without stabilization, and acute suicidal risk. Clients experiencing these conditions need specialized treatment to establish safety and stability before engaging in schema work.

Relative Contraindications require careful assessment and often preparatory work. These include severe trauma with poor emotional regulation, active substance abuse, and certain personality disorders with significant instability. Such conditions don't prevent Schema Therapy but require modifications and additional support.

Risk Factors to monitor include history of self-harm, current life stressors, weak support systems, and previous negative therapy experiences. Clients with these factors need additional safety planning and support resources.

Emotional Regulation Assessment should precede deeper work. Clients need basic skills for managing intense emotions before processing traumatic material. This might require preliminary work on grounding techniques, distress tolerance, and self-soothing strategies.

The case of **Robert** illustrates these safety considerations. Robert, a 30-year-old veteran, sought help for relationship difficulties and anger management. Initial assessment revealed severe PTSD, alcohol abuse, and a history of violence. Rather than immediately beginning schema work, treatment focused first on PTSD stabilization, sobriety support, and anger management skills. Only after six months of preparatory work was Robert ready to explore his underlying schemas safely.

Safety Planning should address potential reactions to schema work. This includes identifying support people, developing coping strategies for intense emotions, and creating action plans for crisis situations. Clients need to know how to contact help if they become overwhelmed outside of sessions.

Pacing Considerations recognize that healing happens gradually. Rushing the process often leads to emotional overwhelm and treatment setbacks. Some clients need months of relationship building and stabilization before tackling core schemas.

Integration with Other Therapeutic Approaches

Schema Therapy's integrative nature allows for seamless combination with other evidence-based treatments. This flexibility enhances treatment effectiveness and allows therapists to address complex presentations requiring multiple interventions.

Cognitive-Behavioral Therapy Integration represents the most natural combination, given Schema Therapy's CBT roots. Traditional CBT techniques like thought records and behavioral experiments can be enhanced with schema awareness. Instead of simply challenging negative thoughts, therapists can help clients understand how these thoughts stem from deeper schema patterns.

Trauma Therapies such as EMDR, CPT, and TF-CBT can be integrated with Schema Therapy for clients with significant trauma histories. Schema work provides the broader context for understanding how traumatic experiences shaped fundamental beliefs and coping patterns. Trauma-specific techniques can address particular incidents while schema work heals the broader patterns that developed in response.

Mindfulness-Based Interventions complement Schema Therapy beautifully. Mindfulness skills help clients observe their schemas and modes without becoming overwhelmed by them. The present-moment awareness cultivated through mindfulness practice supports the healthy adult mode development that is central to schema healing.

Attachment-Based Therapies share significant overlap with Schema Therapy's focus on early relationships and their lasting impact. Techniques from Emotionally Focused Therapy, for example, can be enhanced with schema understanding to address how childhood attachment patterns influence adult relationships.

The case of **Sarah** demonstrates effective integration. Sarah, a 25-year-old graduate student, presented with complex PTSD from childhood sexual abuse, current relationship difficulties, and perfectionist tendencies. Treatment integrated EMDR for specific trauma memories, Schema Therapy for underlying patterns of mistrust and defectiveness, and mindfulness skills for emotional regulation. This combined approach addressed both the specific traumatic experiences and the broader patterns they created.

Family and Couples Therapy Integration recognizes that schemas often play out in close relationships. Understanding each partner's schema profile can illuminate recurring conflicts and provide pathways for healing. Techniques from Gottman Method and Emotionally Focused Therapy can be enhanced with schema awareness to address deeper patterns rather than just surface behaviors.

Group Therapy Integration allows for powerful healing experiences through connection with others who share similar schemas. Group members can provide reality testing, support, and encouragement while practicing new ways of relating. The group becomes a laboratory for healing relationship schemas through corrective interpersonal experiences.

Schema Therapy's flexibility makes it compatible with various theoretical orientations and treatment settings. The key is maintaining the core principles while adapting techniques to fit specific needs and contexts.

Key Insights for Healing

Schema Therapy offers hope for individuals who have struggled with long-standing patterns of emotional difficulty. Unlike approaches that focus solely on symptoms, it addresses the root causes of psychological suffering—the deep beliefs and emotional patterns that formed during our most vulnerable years.

The healing process requires patience, courage, and self-compassion. Schemas developed over years or decades don't change quickly, but they can change. With consistent work and appropriate support, even the most entrenched patterns can be healed, allowing for genuine transformation and the fulfillment of our deepest human needs for connection, safety, and authentic self-expression.

Success in Schema Therapy isn't measured by the absence of all emotional pain, but by the development of healthier patterns of thinking, feeling, and relating. It's about learning to meet our core emotional needs in adaptive ways and developing the internal resources to handle life's inevitable challenges with greater resilience and wisdom.

Chapter 1: Getting Started - Assessment Tools

You can't fix what you can't see clearly. This fundamental truth drives everything we do in Schema Therapy—and nowhere is it more critical than in the assessment phase. Without accurate identification of schemas, their origins, and their current impact, therapy becomes little more than educated guesswork. The five assessment tools presented in this chapter form the bedrock of effective Schema Therapy, providing both therapists and clients with the roadmap needed for successful healing.

Assessment in Schema Therapy goes far beyond simple symptom checklists or diagnostic categories. We're looking for patterns that have shaped an entire lifetime of experience—the deep currents that run beneath the surface of conscious awareness. These patterns don't announce themselves loudly; they hide in the spaces between thoughts, in the assumptions we make about ourselves and others, and in the emotional reactions that seem to come from nowhere.

The genius of Schema Therapy assessment lies in its systematic approach to uncovering these hidden patterns. Each tool serves a specific purpose, building upon the others to create a complete picture of how early experiences continue to shape present-day functioning. This isn't archeological work for its own sake—every piece of information we gather points toward specific interventions and healing strategies.

Exercise 1: Young Schema Questionnaire - Short Form (YSQ-S3)

The Young Schema Questionnaire represents the gold standard for schema identification[9]. This carefully constructed instrument measures the presence and intensity of 18 early maladaptive schemas through 90 specific items. Each item reflects real-world manifestations of schema activity, making the abstract concept of schemas concrete and measurable.

The questionnaire uses a six-point scale ranging from "completely untrue of me" to "describes me perfectly." This scaling allows for nuanced assessment—schemas exist on a continuum rather than as simple present-or-absent categories. A client might score moderately on several schemas while showing severe elevation on one or two primary patterns.

Case Example: Rebecca's Discovery

Rebecca, a 29-year-old nurse, completed the YSQ-S3 during her intake session. Her highest scores emerged on the Unrelenting Standards schema (items like "I must be the best at most of what I do" and "I can't let myself off the hook easily"), the Self-Sacrifice schema (including "I'm so busy doing for the people that I care about, that I have little time for myself"), and the Emotional Deprivation schema ("I feel like I don't have someone to nurture me").

These scores told a clear story. Rebecca had grown up in a household where her mother suffered from chronic depression, leaving Rebecca to care for younger siblings while maintaining perfect grades to earn her father's approval. The YSQ-S3 revealed how these early experiences created three interrelated schemas that now drove her to work double shifts, volunteer for extra responsibilities, and consistently put others' needs before her own.

The questionnaire also revealed surprising elevations on the Vulnerability to Harm schema—something Rebecca hadn't initially recognized. Items like "I worry about being attacked" and "I feel like I have to be very careful about money" reflected an underlying anxiety that pervaded her daily life. This schema connected to her childhood experience of emotional and financial instability, creating a persistent sense of threat that she managed through control and perfectionism.

Administration Guidelines

The YSQ-S3 should be completed in a quiet, private setting where clients can reflect honestly on their experiences. Some clients find the questions emotionally triggering—this reaction itself provides useful clinical information. Explain that the questionnaire measures common human experiences and that elevated scores don't indicate personal failings.

Scoring involves calculating raw scores for each schema domain, then converting these to percentile ranks based on normative data[10]. Scores above the 85th percentile typically indicate clinically significant schema activation, though this should always be interpreted within the broader clinical context.

The questionnaire results guide treatment planning by identifying which schemas require primary attention. Schemas with the highest scores often become the initial focus of therapy, though clinical judgment should consider factors like client readiness and life circumstances.

Exercise 2: Schema Interview Protocol

While the YSQ-S3 provides quantitative data about schema presence, the Schema Interview Protocol offers qualitative depth that brings schemas to life. This structured interview explores the personal history and current manifestations of each schema, creating a rich narrative that both therapist and client can understand.

The protocol follows a systematic format that moves from general life history to specific schema exploration. This approach helps clients connect their current difficulties to their developmental experiences without becoming overwhelmed by traumatic memories early in treatment.

Case Example: Michael's Story

Michael, a 35-year-old IT manager, scored highly on the Abandonment schema during his YSQ-S3 assessment. The Schema Interview Protocol revealed the deeper story behind these scores. Michael's father left when he was six years old, disappearing from his life entirely. His mother, overwhelmed by single parenthood, often threatened to send Michael to live with relatives when he misbehaved.

"I learned early that people leave," Michael explained during the interview. "Even when they say they love you, they can just disappear." The protocol helped uncover how this belief shaped his adult relationships. Michael would become intensely jealous and controlling with romantic partners, constantly seeking reassurance while simultaneously testing their commitment through provocative behavior.

The interview also revealed Michael's coping mechanisms. He had developed an Emotional Inhibition schema as protection against further abandonment—"If I don't let people see how much I need them, they can't hurt me as badly when they leave." This secondary schema actually reinforced his primary abandonment fears by preventing the emotional intimacy that might have contradicted his expectations.

Through careful questioning, the protocol uncovered specific triggers for Michael's abandonment fears: partners arriving home late, changes in their tone of voice, or any mention of other relationships. These triggers would activate his schema, flooding him with the terror of that six-year-old boy whose father never came home.

Interview Structure and Techniques

The protocol begins with broad developmental history, allowing clients to tell their story without immediate focus on pathology. Questions like "What was your family like when you were growing up?" and "How did your parents show love and affection?" open conversations naturally.

As specific schemas emerge, the interview becomes more targeted. For each identified schema, explore three key areas: developmental origins (how did this pattern develop?), current manifestations (how does it show up today?), and coping responses (what do you do when this schema gets activated?).

Effective interviewing requires balancing structure with flexibility. While the protocol provides a framework, follow the client's natural flow of associations. Often, the most important information emerges in seemingly tangential comments or emotional reactions.

Pay attention to both content and process during the interview. How does the client tell their story? Do they minimize trauma or become emotionally overwhelmed? These reactions provide information about their coping styles and readiness for deeper work.

Exercise 3: Childhood Experiences Timeline

Visual representations of life experiences can reveal patterns that purely verbal processing might miss. The Childhood Experiences Timeline creates a concrete map of significant events, relationships, and developmental milestones that shaped schema formation.

This exercise involves creating a chronological representation of childhood experiences from birth through adolescence. Clients identify both positive and negative events, noting their emotional impact and any lasting effects on their beliefs about themselves and others.

Case Example: Patricia's Pattern Recognition

Patricia, a 41-year-old attorney, initially described her childhood as "normal" with "typical family problems." Her timeline revealed a different picture. From ages 3-7, her timeline showed repeated hospitalizations for severe asthma, during which she felt abandoned and terrified. Ages 8-12 were marked by her parents' volatile relationship, culminating in a bitter divorce that left Patricia feeling responsible for holding the family together.

The timeline's visual format helped Patricia recognize patterns she'd never connected before. Each major stressor in her childhood was followed by increased responsibility and pressure to be "strong" for others. She could see how her Unrelenting Standards and Self-Sacrifice schemas developed as adaptations to these overwhelming circumstances.

Most significantly, the timeline revealed that Patricia's schemas didn't develop in isolation. Her perfectionism (Unrelenting Standards) served to prevent the chaos she experienced during her parents' fighting. Her self-sacrifice protected her from the guilt she felt about her parents' divorce. The visual representation showed how these schemas formed an interconnected system designed to manage overwhelming emotional experiences.

The timeline also highlighted positive experiences that Patricia had forgotten or minimized. Her relationship with her grandmother provided periods of unconditional love and acceptance that contradicted her dominant schemas. Recognizing these positive experiences became important for accessing her Healthy Adult mode later in treatment.

Construction Guidelines

Use a large sheet of paper or poster board divided into age ranges (0-3, 4-7, 8-12, 13-18). Encourage clients to include various types of experiences: family events, school experiences, friendships, medical issues, moves, losses, and achievements.

Different colors can represent different types of experiences—red for traumatic events, blue for losses, green for positive experiences, yellow for achievements. This color coding helps patterns become visually apparent.

Encourage clients to note their emotional responses to events, not just the events themselves. How did they feel during their parents' divorce? What did they tell themselves when Dad left? These internal responses often reveal schema formation in progress.

The timeline should include both major events and ongoing patterns. A father's emotional unavailability might not be a single event but a chronic reality that shaped schema development over years.

Exercise 4: Core Emotional Needs Assessment

15

Human beings enter the world with universal emotional needs that must be met for healthy development[11]. The Core Emotional Needs Assessment identifies which of these fundamental needs were unmet during childhood, providing direct links to specific schema formation.

The assessment examines seven core need areas: safety and stability, nurturance and affection, acceptance and praise, empathy and understanding, guidance and protection, validation of feelings and needs, and encouragement of autonomy and independence. For each area, clients rate how well their needs were met during different developmental periods.

Case Example: Jonathan's Needs Analysis

Jonathan, a 26-year-old graduate student, struggled with social anxiety and feelings of inadequacy. His Core Emotional Needs Assessment revealed profound unmet needs in the areas of acceptance and validation. His parents, both high-achieving professionals, provided material security but little emotional support.

"I got praise when I succeeded, but I never felt accepted for who I was," Jonathan reflected. "Everything was conditional on performance." The assessment showed how his need for unconditional acceptance went unmet, leading to the development of a Defectiveness schema—a belief that something was fundamentally wrong with him.

The assessment also revealed unmet needs for empathy and understanding. Jonathan's parents responded to his emotional distress with advice or criticism rather than comfort. "They meant well, but they never just listened," he noted. This pattern created an Emotional Deprivation schema that left Jonathan feeling fundamentally alone and misunderstood.

Interestingly, Jonathan's needs for guidance and protection were adequately met. His parents provided clear rules and kept him physically safe. This explained why his schemas centered on emotional rather than safety concerns—he developed beliefs about his worth and lovability rather than about physical danger.

16

The assessment helped Jonathan understand that his difficulties weren't character flaws but natural responses to unmet developmental needs. This realization reduced his shame and opened pathways for healing focused on getting those needs met in healthier ways.

Assessment Implementation

Present the needs assessment as an exploration rather than a test. Each need area includes specific questions about childhood experiences. For safety and stability: "Did you feel secure and protected in your home?" For nurturance: "Did you receive adequate physical affection and comfort?"

Use a rating scale from 1 (needs rarely met) to 5 (needs consistently met). Encourage clients to consider different developmental periods, as needs fulfillment often changes over time. A parent might provide excellent nurturing during early childhood but become emotionally unavailable during adolescence.

Discuss the results collaboratively, helping clients connect unmet needs to current difficulties. This connection should feel enlightening rather than blaming—the goal is understanding, not fault-finding.

The assessment results guide treatment planning by identifying which emotional needs require attention in therapy. The therapeutic relationship itself becomes a vehicle for meeting previously unmet needs in age-appropriate ways.

Exercise 5: Schema Severity Rating Scale

Not all schemas carry equal weight in a person's psychological functioning. The Schema Severity Rating Scale helps prioritize treatment by assessing three dimensions: frequency of activation, intensity of emotional response, and life impact of each identified schema.

This tool moves beyond simple presence or absence to examine how schemas actually function in daily life. A schema might be present but dormant, activated only under specific circumstances. Another schema might be constantly active but create relatively minor disruption. Still others might be occasionally triggered but create overwhelming emotional responses when activated.

Case Example: Lisa's Schema Hierarchy

Lisa, a 33-year-old marketing director, showed elevated scores on multiple schemas during assessment. The Severity Rating Scale helped prioritize which schemas required immediate attention. Her Unrelenting Standards schema received high scores on all three dimensions—it activated daily (frequency), created intense anxiety and self-criticism (intensity), and significantly impacted her work performance and relationships (life impact).

Her Abandonment schema, while also present, showed a different pattern. It activated less frequently but with extreme intensity during relationship conflicts. The life impact was moderate because Lisa had learned to avoid situations that triggered these fears. This information suggested that Unrelenting Standards should receive primary treatment focus, with Abandonment addressed as it emerged in the therapeutic relationship.

Lisa's Emotional Inhibition schema showed yet another pattern—high frequency but lower intensity and moderate life impact. She consistently suppressed emotional expression but had developed effective coping mechanisms that minimized disruption. This schema could be addressed later in treatment when she had more emotional regulation skills.

The rating scale revealed that Lisa's schemas worked together as an interconnected system. Her perfectionism (Unrelenting Standards) protected against criticism that might trigger abandonment fears. Her emotional inhibition prevented the vulnerability that perfectionism couldn't control. Understanding these connections helped prioritize interventions that would create positive cascading effects across multiple schemas.

Rating Methodology

For each identified schema, clients rate three dimensions on a scale of 1-10. Frequency measures how often the schema gets activated—daily, weekly, monthly, or only under specific circumstances. Intensity assesses the emotional impact when the schema is triggered—mild discomfort to overwhelming distress. Life impact examines how much the schema interferes with work, relationships, and overall functioning.

Total severity scores (frequency + intensity + life impact) provide a quantitative basis for treatment prioritization. Schemas with scores above 21 typically require immediate attention, while those scoring 15-21 might be addressed secondarily.

The scale should be administered after other assessment tools provide clear schema identification. Clients need to understand their schemas before they can accurately rate their impact.

Consider readministering the scale periodically during treatment to track progress. As primary schemas heal, secondary schemas may become more prominent or other schemas may emerge as defenses are reduced.

Building Your Assessment Foundation

These five assessment tools work together to create a complete picture of schema functioning. The YSQ-S3 provides standardized measurement of schema presence. The Schema Interview Protocol adds personal narrative and developmental context. The Childhood Experiences Timeline visually maps schema origins. The Core Emotional Needs Assessment identifies the fundamental gaps that created schemas. The Schema Severity Rating Scale prioritizes treatment focus.

Effective assessment requires patience and skill. Rush the process, and you'll miss critical information. Take too long, and clients may become overwhelmed or lose motivation. The goal is creating a collaborative understanding that feels both accurate and hopeful—

accurate enough to guide effective treatment, hopeful enough to maintain engagement.

Good assessment also normalizes the client's experience. Schemas aren't character defects; they're understandable adaptations to difficult circumstances. The child who developed a Mistrust schema in response to abuse was being smart, not pathological. The adult who maintains this schema may need help updating their protective strategies, but the original adaptation deserves respect.

Assessment findings should always be presented with compassion and hope. Yes, these patterns have created difficulties, but they can be changed. Yes, the origins may be painful, but healing is possible. The assessment process itself begins the therapeutic work by creating new ways of understanding old problems.

Essential Elements for Success

Several key principles guide effective schema assessment. First, maintain curiosity rather than certainty. Schemas are complex, and initial impressions may prove incomplete or incorrect. Stay open to new information and revised understandings as therapy progresses.

Second, balance thoroughness with sensitivity. Some clients need extensive assessment to feel understood and ready for treatment. Others become overwhelmed by too much initial focus on their difficulties. Adjust your approach based on the client's capacity and preferences.

Third, connect assessment findings to treatment possibilities. Don't just identify problems; point toward solutions. Help clients see how understanding their schemas opens pathways for change that weren't visible before.

Key Learning Points

- Assessment forms the foundation for all effective Schema Therapy interventions

- Multiple tools provide different but complementary information about schema functioning
- The YSQ-S3 offers standardized measurement while interview protocols provide personal context
- Visual timelines help clients recognize patterns they might otherwise miss
- Core needs assessment directly links childhood experiences to current difficulties
- Severity ratings guide treatment prioritization and resource allocation
- Effective assessment balances thoroughness with client emotional capacity
- Assessment findings should be presented with both accuracy and hope for change

Chapter 2: Schema Identification and Awareness

Awareness is the first step toward freedom. You can't change what you don't see, and you can't see what you haven't learned to recognize. Schemas operate like background programs on a computer— constantly running, influencing everything, but invisible to the user. The exercises in this chapter bring these hidden patterns into the light of conscious awareness, creating the foundation for all healing work that follows.

Schema identification goes beyond simply knowing which patterns affect you. True awareness involves understanding how these patterns show up in daily life, what triggers them, how they feel in your body, and how they connect to your personal history. This chapter provides seven practical tools that build schema awareness from multiple angles, creating a complete picture of how these deep patterns shape your experience.

The beauty of these exercises lies in their practicality. They don't require years of therapy or advanced psychological training. They simply require honesty, curiosity, and the willingness to look at yourself with both compassion and clarity. Each exercise builds on the others, creating layers of understanding that make schemas impossible to ignore—and therefore possible to change.

Exercise 6: Schema Flashcards

Quick Reference Cards for Schema Recognition

Schema flashcards serve as portable awareness tools that help you identify schema activation in real-time. Each card contains a schema name, its core belief, common triggers, typical emotional reactions, and behavioral patterns. Think of them as field guides for your inner world—reference materials that help you name what you're experiencing as it happens.

The power of flashcards lies in their immediacy. Schema activation often happens quickly and subtly. You might feel suddenly anxious in a meeting, inexplicably angry at your partner, or mysteriously depressed after a social gathering. Flashcards help you connect these reactions to their underlying schema patterns before the moment passes.

Case Example: Thomas and His Perfectionist Trap

Thomas, a 34-year-old architect, created flashcards after identifying Unrelenting Standards as his primary schema. His card read: "Core belief: I must be perfect or I'm worthless. Triggers: Making mistakes, receiving criticism, comparing myself to others. Feelings: Anxiety, shame, frustration. Behaviors: Working excessive hours, avoiding tasks where I might fail, being critical of others."

During a team meeting where his design received minor criticism, Thomas felt his chest tighten and his mind race with self-attacking thoughts. He excused himself briefly and consulted his flashcard. Seeing his pattern written clearly helped him recognize the schema activation instead of getting lost in it. "This is my Unrelenting Standards schema," he told himself. "The criticism doesn't mean I'm worthless—it means I'm human."

The flashcard helped Thomas respond differently than usual. Instead of staying late to completely redesign the project (his typical overcompensation), he made reasonable revisions and went home at normal time. Over months of using the cards, Thomas developed the ability to catch schema activation earlier and respond more healthily.

Creating Effective Flashcards

Each flashcard should include five key elements: schema name, core belief statement, common triggers, typical emotional reactions, and behavioral patterns. Keep language simple and personal—use your own words to describe how the schema shows up in your life.

Make cards small enough to carry easily but large enough to read comfortably. Index cards work well, or you can create digital versions

23

on your phone. Some people prefer different colors for different schema types—red for abandonment fears, blue for perfectionism, green for people-pleasing patterns.

Include coping reminders on each card. What helps you when this schema gets activated? Thomas added: "Breathe deeply. This feeling will pass. Good enough is often good enough. I am worthy regardless of my performance."

Update your cards as your understanding deepens. Early versions might focus on recognition, while later versions include more sophisticated coping strategies and healthy responses.

Exercise 7: Personal Schema Diary

Daily Tracking of Schema Activation

The Personal Schema Diary creates a systematic record of how schemas show up in daily life. This ongoing documentation reveals patterns that single incidents might miss—the specific times of day when certain schemas activate, the relationships that trigger particular patterns, or the life circumstances that make you more vulnerable to schema flooding.

Think of the diary as scientific research into your own psychological patterns. You're gathering data about when, where, and how your schemas operate. This information becomes the foundation for targeted interventions and healing strategies.

Case Example: Maria's Abandonment Patterns

Maria, a 28-year-old teacher, kept a schema diary focusing on her Abandonment schema. Her entries revealed surprising patterns. The schema activated most strongly on Sunday evenings when she anticipated the work week ahead. It also triggered whenever her boyfriend didn't respond to texts within an hour, when friends made plans without including her, or when she saw social media posts of others having fun.

One typical entry read: "Sunday 7 PM - Boyfriend went home after weekend together. Immediate panic that he's losing interest. Checked phone 12 times waiting for his 'got home safely' text. Felt like that little girl again when Dad would leave for business trips. Called Sarah for reassurance, but felt pathetic afterward."

The diary helped Maria recognize that her Abandonment schema had specific triggers (separations, delayed responses, exclusion) and predictable patterns (checking behaviors, seeking reassurance, shame spirals). More importantly, it showed her that these reactions were schema-driven rather than reality-based. Her boyfriend consistently returned her calls and made plans with her—the threat of abandonment was in her schema, not in their relationship.

After three months of diary keeping, Maria could predict when her schema would activate and prepare coping strategies. Sunday evenings became opportunities for self-care rather than panic sessions.

Diary Structure and Implementation

Each diary entry should include date and time, the situation or trigger, which schema activated, emotional reactions, physical sensations, thoughts or beliefs that arose, behavioral responses, and effectiveness of any coping strategies used.

Keep entries brief but specific. Instead of "felt bad after work," write "felt inadequate after boss gave feedback on my presentation— Defectiveness schema activated with thoughts that I'm not smart enough for this job."

Look for patterns across entries. Do certain schemas activate more on specific days? In particular relationships? During certain seasons or life circumstances? These patterns reveal important information about your schema functioning.

Rate the intensity of schema activation on a scale of 1-10. This helps track progress over time and identifies which triggers create the strongest reactions.

Exercise 8: Schema Triggers Identification

Mapping Situations That Activate Specific Schemas

Schema triggers are the external events, internal thoughts, or interpersonal situations that activate your schema patterns. Identifying these triggers with precision gives you the power to prepare for difficult situations and respond more consciously when they occur.

Triggers often fall into predictable categories: interpersonal (relationship conflicts, criticism, rejection), environmental (stressful work situations, financial pressure, health concerns), internal (negative self-talk, memories, physical sensations), or temporal (anniversaries, holidays, developmental milestones).

Case Example: David's Mistrust Schema Mapping

David, a 42-year-old consultant, mapped the triggers for his Mistrust/Abuse schema after recognizing how it damaged his business relationships. His trigger map revealed several categories: new client meetings (fear of being taken advantage of), contract negotiations (anticipating deception), team collaborations (expecting betrayal), and social events (scanning for signs of manipulation).

More subtle triggers included people being overly friendly (suspicion of hidden agendas), receiving unexpected compliments (searching for ulterior motives), and partners changing plans (interpreting as evidence of lies). David realized his schema created a constant state of hypervigilance that exhausted him and pushed people away.

The mapping exercise revealed that his triggers often involved situations where he had less control or where others' motivations weren't completely transparent. This awareness helped David develop specific strategies for each trigger category. For new client meetings, he prepared by reminding himself that most people are trustworthy and that his skepticism, while protective, could damage potential relationships.

David also discovered positive triggers—situations that activated his Healthy Adult mode. These included working with long-term clients who had proven their reliability, collaborating with his business partner who had consistently demonstrated integrity, and spending time with his sister who had never betrayed his trust. Recognizing these positive triggers helped David seek out situations that supported his healing rather than reinforced his schema.

Creating Your Trigger Map

Start by listing situations where you've noticed schema activation. Include both obvious triggers (being criticized for Defectiveness schema) and subtle ones (seeing happy couples for Emotional Deprivation schema).

Organize triggers into categories that make sense for your experience. Common categories include relationship triggers, work triggers, family triggers, health triggers, financial triggers, and anniversary triggers.

Rate each trigger's intensity from 1-10. Some triggers might create mild schema activation while others cause overwhelming reactions. Understanding intensity helps you prepare appropriate coping strategies.

Identify the early warning signs for each trigger. What thoughts, feelings, or physical sensations signal that a schema is becoming activated? The earlier you can catch activation, the more options you have for responding consciously.

Exercise 9: Schema Beliefs Inventory

Cataloging Maladaptive Core Beliefs

Schemas express themselves through specific beliefs about yourself, others, and the world. The Schema Beliefs Inventory systematically identifies these core beliefs, creating a catalog of the automatic thoughts that drive emotional reactions and behavioral choices.

These beliefs often operate outside conscious awareness, functioning as background assumptions that shape perception and interpretation. Making them explicit allows you to examine their accuracy and helpfulness in your current life circumstances.

Case Example: Jennifer's Defectiveness Beliefs

Jennifer, a 31-year-old nurse, created a beliefs inventory for her Defectiveness schema. Her catalog included: "Something is fundamentally wrong with me," "If people really knew me, they would reject me," "I have to hide my true self to be accepted," "Other people are more worthy of love than I am," "My needs and feelings don't matter," and "I don't deserve good things in life."

Reading these beliefs together was shocking for Jennifer. "I never realized how harsh and absolute these thoughts were," she reflected. "No wonder I feel so bad about myself—I'm constantly telling myself these terrible things."

The inventory helped Jennifer recognize how these beliefs influenced her daily choices. She avoided social situations where people might "discover" her flaws. She stayed in an unfulfilling job because she believed she didn't deserve better. She tolerated poor treatment from others because she thought she wasn't worthy of respect.

Creating the inventory was the first step toward challenging these beliefs. Jennifer began questioning each one: "Is it really true that something is fundamentally wrong with me? What evidence supports this belief? What evidence contradicts it? How would I talk to a friend who told me they believed these things about themselves?"

Building Your Beliefs Inventory

For each identified schema, list the specific beliefs it generates. Start with core beliefs about yourself (I am...), then beliefs about others (People are...), and finally beliefs about the world (Life is...).

Use your natural language rather than clinical terminology. How do you actually talk to yourself when the schema is active? What assumptions do you make about other people's motivations?

Include both global beliefs (I'm worthless) and specific situational beliefs (If I make a mistake at work, everyone will think I'm incompetent). Both types influence your emotional reactions and behavioral choices.

Notice the absoluteness of schema-driven beliefs. They often include words like "always," "never," "everyone," "no one," "completely," or "totally." This all-or-nothing thinking is a hallmark of schema activation.

Exercise 10: Early Memory Exploration

Connecting Childhood Experiences to Current Schemas

Early memories hold the keys to understanding how your schemas developed. The Early Memory Exploration exercise systematically examines formative experiences to create direct connections between past events and present patterns.

This isn't archeological work for its own sake—understanding origins helps you recognize that your schemas made sense given your childhood circumstances. They were smart adaptations to difficult situations, not character flaws or evidence of your inadequacy.

Case Example: Michael's Abandonment Origins

Michael, a 39-year-old sales manager, explored early memories related to his Abandonment schema. His most powerful memory involved being seven years old and waiting at school for his mother to pick him up. She was two hours late, and he sat alone on the steps, convinced she had forgotten him or something terrible had happened.

"I felt so small and scared," Michael recalled. "I made up stories about where she might be, and all of them involved her being hurt or dead. When she finally arrived, she was angry that I was crying instead of relieved that I was safe."

This memory revealed the origin of Michael's belief that people he loved would disappear without warning. His child mind had concluded that loved ones were unreliable and that his emotional reactions were burdensome to others. These beliefs became the foundation of his Abandonment schema.

Exploring additional memories revealed a pattern: his mother was often overwhelmed and unpredictable, sometimes loving and attentive, other times distracted and unavailable. Young Michael developed hypervigilance about signs that people were losing interest in him—a survival strategy that protected him from repeated disappointment.

Understanding these origins helped Michael develop compassion for his schema rather than shame. That seven-year-old boy had been smart to develop strategies for managing an unpredictable caregiver. The adult Michael could appreciate that protection while updating his strategies for current relationships.

Memory Exploration Guidelines

Focus on memories that carry strong emotional charges rather than just significant events. The feelings attached to memories often matter more than the objective details of what happened.

Look for patterns across multiple memories rather than focusing on single incidents. Schemas typically develop from repeated experiences rather than one-time traumas.

Include both obvious memories (divorce, abuse, neglect) and subtle ones (emotional unavailability, conditional love, being treated as an adult too young). Sometimes the absence of needed experiences is as important as the presence of harmful ones.

Pay attention to the decisions your child-self made about these experiences. What conclusions did you draw about yourself, others, and relationships? These childhood decisions often become adult schemas.

Exercise 11: Schema Body Scan

Identifying Physical Sensations Associated with Schemas

Schemas don't just live in your thoughts—they express themselves through physical sensations, muscle tension, breathing patterns, and nervous system activation. The Schema Body Scan helps you recognize these somatic markers, creating another avenue for early detection and intervention.

Your body often recognizes schema activation before your mind does. Learning to read these physical signals gives you earlier warning and more time to respond consciously rather than reactively.

Case Example: Sarah's Anxiety Embodiment

Sarah, a 26-year-old graduate student, learned to recognize how her Vulnerability to Harm schema showed up in her body. During the body scan exercise, she noticed that anticipating negative events created specific physical patterns: tightness in her chest, shallow breathing, clenched jaw, and cold hands.

"It's like my whole body goes into alarm mode," Sarah observed. "My shoulders creep up toward my ears, and I feel like I'm bracing for impact even when nothing threatening is actually happening."

Sarah discovered that her body held the memory of childhood medical trauma—multiple surgeries and hospitalizations that had left her feeling fragile and vulnerable. Her nervous system had learned to scan constantly for signs of danger, creating chronic muscle tension and hypervigilance.

The body scan helped Sarah develop early intervention strategies. When she noticed the familiar chest tightness, she could use breathing exercises to calm her nervous system before anxiety spiraled out of

31

control. When her shoulders began rising, she could consciously relax them and remind herself that she was safe in the present moment.

Over time, Sarah learned to trust her body's wisdom while not being controlled by its alarm systems. Her physical sensations became information rather than commands, helping her respond more skillfully to real and imagined threats.

Conducting Effective Body Scans

Find a quiet space where you can sit or lie comfortably without interruption. Close your eyes and take several slow, deep breaths to settle into your body.

Start at the top of your head and slowly move your attention down through your body: forehead, eyes, jaw, neck, shoulders, arms, chest, back, abdomen, hips, legs, and feet. Notice any areas of tension, tightness, numbness, or unusual sensations.

When you find areas of tension or discomfort, pause and explore them gently. What does this sensation feel like? How long has it been there? What emotions or thoughts arise when you focus on this area?

Connect physical sensations to schema patterns. Does chest tightness correspond to abandonment fears? Do clenched fists relate to anger from your Self-Sacrifice schema? These connections help you recognize schema activation through body awareness.

Exercise 12: Schema Genogram

Family Patterns and Intergenerational Transmission

Schemas don't develop in isolation—they're often passed down through families like heirlooms, sometimes for generations. The Schema Genogram maps these family patterns, helping you understand how the schemas that affect you may have affected your parents, grandparents, and other relatives.

This exercise isn't about blaming your family or excusing your difficulties. It's about understanding the larger context in which your schemas developed and recognizing the intergenerational patterns that may require conscious intervention to change.

Case Example: Robert's Family Legacy

Robert, a 45-year-old engineer, created a genogram for his family's Emotional Inhibition patterns. The map revealed three generations of men who struggled to express feelings openly. His grandfather, a World War II veteran, had returned from combat emotionally shut down and never spoke about his experiences. Robert's father had learned that "real men don't cry" and had passed this message to Robert and his brothers.

The genogram showed how trauma and cultural messages had combined to create a family legacy of emotional suppression. Robert's grandfather's survival mechanism (emotional numbness in response to combat trauma) became a family rule that affected subsequent generations, even though they hadn't experienced the original trauma.

Understanding this pattern helped Robert develop compassion for his family's emotional limitations while choosing to break the cycle with his own children. "My grandfather did what he needed to do to survive the war," Robert reflected. "My father did what he learned from his father. Now I can choose something different for my kids."

The genogram also revealed family strengths that could support Robert's healing. His grandmother had been emotionally expressive and nurturing, providing a model for healthy emotional connection. His sister had learned to balance emotional expression with appropriate boundaries. These positive patterns gave Robert hope and practical examples for his own growth.

Creating Your Family Genogram

Start with a basic family tree going back at least three generations. Include parents, grandparents, siblings, aunts, uncles, and significant others who influenced family dynamics.

For each family member, note relevant information: major life events, personality characteristics, mental health struggles, relationship patterns, coping mechanisms, and any known traumas or significant stressors.

Identify patterns that repeat across generations. Do family members struggle with similar issues? Are there recurring themes in how relationships are handled, emotions are expressed, or stress is managed?

Use different colors or symbols to represent different schemas or patterns. You might use red for abandonment issues, blue for perfectionism, green for emotional inhibition, and so on.

Look for both negative patterns you want to change and positive patterns you want to strengthen. Every family has both destructive and healing elements—the goal is understanding which patterns serve you and which ones need updating.

Stepping Into Greater Awareness

Schema awareness isn't a destination—it's an ongoing practice that deepens over time. The exercises in this chapter provide multiple pathways for recognizing how your deepest patterns show up in daily life. Some people connect most easily with cognitive approaches like belief inventories. Others respond better to somatic awareness through body scans. Still others find family patterns most illuminating.

Use all these tools to create a complete picture of your schema functioning. Each exercise reveals different aspects of the same underlying patterns, building a robust understanding that can't be shaken by momentary doubts or temporary setbacks.

Schema awareness often brings initial discomfort as you recognize how these patterns have influenced your life. This discomfort is normal and temporary—the price of admission to greater freedom and choice. Once you can see your schemas clearly, you're no longer at their mercy. You can work with them instead of being controlled by them.

The real gift of awareness is choice. You can't choose what happened to you in childhood, but you can choose how you respond to those experiences today. You can't eliminate your schemas entirely, but you can change your relationship to them. Awareness makes all of this possible.

Chapter 3: Schema Mode Mapping and Management

Your internal world contains multiple parts, each with its own voice, needs, and ways of responding to life's challenges. Schema Mode Theory recognizes this multiplicity, providing a framework for understanding the different aspects of yourself that become active in various situations[12]. Unlike schemas, which are relatively stable traits, modes are temporary states that shift throughout the day based on what you encounter and how you interpret it.

Think of modes as different characters in your internal drama—each with its own costume, script, and motivation. Sometimes your Vulnerable Child mode takes center stage, feeling small and frightened in the face of criticism. Other times your Demanding Parent mode dominates, pushing yourself and others toward impossible standards. Healthy functioning involves having access to all parts while allowing your Healthy Adult mode to serve as the wise director of this internal theater.

The exercises in this chapter help you recognize these different parts, understand when and why they become active, and develop the skills to strengthen your Healthy Adult mode while caring for the wounded parts that need attention. This work is both profoundly healing and immediately practical—once you understand your modes, you can respond to life's challenges with greater flexibility and wisdom.

Exercise 13: Mode Identification Checklist

Recognizing the 17 Different Schema Modes

Mode identification begins with learning to recognize the distinct emotional states and behavioral patterns that characterize each mode. The 17 schema modes fall into four main categories: Child modes (Vulnerable Child, Angry Child, Impulsive Child, Happy Child), Dysfunctional Parent modes (Punitive Parent, Demanding Parent),

Coping modes (Compliant Surrenderer, Detached Protector, Overcompensator), and the Healthy Adult mode[13].

Each mode has its own voice, emotional tone, and typical behaviors. Learning to identify which mode is active at any given moment provides crucial information about what you need and how to respond most effectively.

Case Example: Rachel's Mode Discovery

Rachel, a 32-year-old marketing director, completed the mode identification checklist and was surprised to discover how frequently she shifted between different parts of herself. Her Vulnerable Child mode showed up whenever she received criticism at work, leaving her feeling small, inadequate, and desperate for reassurance. This part of her wanted to hide under her desk and cry.

Her Demanding Parent mode activated when she felt threatened or overwhelmed, driving her to work 12-hour days and criticize team members for not meeting her impossible standards. This voice told her that anything less than perfection was failure and that she needed to control every detail to prevent disaster.

When overwhelmed by these competing demands, Rachel would shift into Detached Protector mode, becoming emotionally numb and going through the motions of work and relationships without genuine engagement. This part protected her from feeling too much but also cut her off from joy, creativity, and meaningful connection.

Rachel's Happy Child mode rarely appeared, emerging only during rare moments of play with her nieces or while painting in her spare time. This part of her was spontaneous, curious, and alive—qualities that had been largely suppressed by the demands of her other modes.

The checklist helped Rachel understand that these weren't random mood swings but predictable responses to specific triggers. Her Vulnerable Child activated when she felt criticized or rejected. Her Demanding Parent took over when she felt out of control. Her

Detached Protector emerged when emotions became too intense to handle.

Using the Identification Checklist

The checklist includes specific behavioral and emotional indicators for each mode. For Vulnerable Child mode, these might include feeling small or helpless, wanting comfort and reassurance, or having difficulty making decisions. For Demanding Parent mode, indicators include harsh self-criticism, perfectionist demands, or impatience with others' mistakes.

Rate how frequently you experience each mode on a scale from 1 (never) to 5 (very often). This creates a profile of your most and least active modes, helping prioritize which modes need attention.

Pay attention to transitions between modes. What triggers cause you to shift from one mode to another? Understanding these transitions helps you anticipate mode changes and respond more consciously.

Notice which modes feel most comfortable or familiar. Often, our dominant coping modes feel "normal" because we've used them for so long, even though they may not serve our current needs effectively.

Exercise 14: Daily Mode Tracking

Monitoring Mode Shifts Throughout the Day

Daily mode tracking creates real-time awareness of how your internal states shift in response to different situations, relationships, and stressors. This exercise reveals patterns that might be invisible during single therapy sessions or isolated self-reflection periods.

The tracking process itself often becomes therapeutic, creating space between your experience and your reaction to it. When you can observe your modes objectively, you're less likely to be completely taken over by them.

Case Example: James's Work Day Patterns

James, a 38-year-old teacher, tracked his modes for two weeks and discovered surprising patterns. His mornings typically began in Healthy Adult mode—he felt capable, centered, and ready for the day. However, his first challenging student interaction would often trigger his Vulnerable Child mode, leaving him feeling incompetent and overwhelmed.

This vulnerability would quickly activate his Demanding Parent mode as he tried to regain control. He'd become harsh with students, set unrealistic expectations for lesson plans, and berate himself for any perceived failures. By lunch time, the stress of maintaining these demanding standards would push him into Detached Protector mode, where he'd go through the motions of teaching while feeling emotionally disconnected from his students and colleagues.

James's tracking revealed that Friday afternoons were particularly difficult. The accumulated stress of the week, combined with exhaustion, made him more vulnerable to mode flipping. He also noticed that certain students consistently triggered his modes—particularly those who reminded him of himself as an anxious, approval-seeking child.

The tracking helped James develop targeted interventions. He began starting difficult conversations with students from his Healthy Adult mode, taking time to center himself before responding to challenging behaviors. He scheduled brief mindfulness breaks between classes to prevent mode accumulation throughout the day.

Implementing Daily Tracking

Create a simple tracking sheet with hourly time slots and space to note which mode was most active, what triggered any mode shifts, and how you responded. Use shorthand notation to make tracking quick and sustainable—VC for Vulnerable Child, DP for Demanding Parent, HA for Healthy Adult.

Set reminder alerts on your phone to check in with yourself several times throughout the day. The goal isn't perfect accuracy but developing the habit of internal awareness.

Note the intensity of mode activation on a scale of 1-10. Sometimes modes are barely perceptible, while other times they completely dominate your experience.

Look for patterns across days and weeks. Do certain times of day, people, or situations consistently trigger specific modes? Are there protective factors that help you maintain Healthy Adult functioning?

Exercise 15: Mode Dialogue Scripts

Conversations Between Different Modes

Mode dialogue scripts create structured conversations between different parts of yourself, allowing each mode to express its needs, concerns, and perspectives. This internal diplomacy often reveals conflicts between modes and helps develop more harmonious relationships between different aspects of yourself.

These dialogues aren't just intellectual exercises—they're opportunities for genuine internal healing and integration. Often, conflicting modes represent different ages and stages of development, each carrying important information about your needs and fears.

Case Example: Susan's Internal Negotiation

Susan, a 29-year-old lawyer, used mode dialogues to address the conflict between her Vulnerable Child and Demanding Parent modes. Her Vulnerable Child felt overwhelmed by work demands and wanted comfort and reassurance. Her Demanding Parent insisted that she work harder and criticized her for any signs of weakness or need.

In a typical dialogue, her Vulnerable Child might say: "I'm so tired and scared. Everyone expects so much from me, and I don't think I can do it. I just want someone to take care of me and tell me everything will be okay."

Her Demanding Parent would respond: "You can't be weak like this. Successful people don't whine about being tired. You need to work harder and stop being so needy. Other people are counting on you, and you can't let them down."

Through facilitated dialogue work, Susan helped these parts begin talking to each other more compassionately. Her Healthy Adult mode learned to mediate these conversations, helping both parts feel heard while finding realistic solutions.

The Healthy Adult might say to the Vulnerable Child: "I hear that you're feeling overwhelmed and scared. Those feelings make sense given how hard you're working. You deserve comfort and support." To the Demanding Parent: "I appreciate how much you care about success and helping others. Your drive and determination are real strengths."

Then, finding a middle path: "What if we worked really hard during work hours but made sure to rest and recharge in the evenings? We can be successful without sacrificing our basic needs for comfort and connection."

Creating Effective Mode Dialogues

Start by identifying the two modes that seem most in conflict or that create the most internal tension. Give each mode a voice and let them express their perspectives fully before trying to find solutions.

Use different chairs or positions for each mode to make the dialogue more experiential. Physically moving between positions helps access the different emotional states more fully.

Let each mode speak in its natural voice and language. The Vulnerable Child might use simple, emotional language, while the Demanding Parent might be more harsh and absolute in its statements.

41

Bring in the Healthy Adult mode as a mediator once both sides have been heard. The Healthy Adult can acknowledge the valid concerns of each mode while finding balanced solutions that meet everyone's needs.

Exercise 16: Mode Intensity Rating

Measuring the Strength of Mode Activation

Mode intensity varies dramatically based on triggers, stress levels, and current life circumstances. The same mode that creates mild discomfort on a good day might completely overwhelm you during periods of high stress or vulnerability. Learning to assess and track mode intensity helps you calibrate your responses and choose appropriate coping strategies.

Intensity rating also helps you recognize when modes are becoming problematic. Mild activation of your Demanding Parent mode might actually be helpful for motivation and achievement. Severe activation might create perfectionist paralysis or damage relationships through impossible expectations.

Case Example: Mark's Anger Escalation

Mark, a 35-year-old sales manager, learned to rate the intensity of his Angry Child mode to prevent explosive episodes that damaged his relationships. He developed a 1-10 scale where 1-3 represented mild irritation that he could manage easily, 4-6 indicated significant anger that required active coping strategies, and 7-10 meant overwhelming rage that often led to regrettable actions.

Mark discovered that his Angry Child mode had specific escalation patterns. It would start at level 2-3 when he felt dismissed or criticized. If he didn't address these feelings early, they would build to level 5-6 when he'd become sarcastic and passive-aggressive. At level 7-8, he'd start yelling or saying hurtful things. Level 9-10 episodes involved complete loss of control with potential for verbal or physical aggression.

The intensity rating system helped Mark intervene earlier in the escalation process. At level 3-4, he could use breathing exercises and brief time-outs to prevent further escalation. At level 5-6, he needed more active strategies like physical exercise or calling a friend for support. Once he reached level 7 or above, his only effective strategy was complete removal from the triggering situation until he could calm down.

Mark also learned to recognize the physical signs of increasing intensity: muscle tension at level 3, rapid heartbeat at level 5, and feeling hot or dizzy at level 7. These somatic markers gave him additional early warning signals for mode escalation.

Developing Your Intensity Scale

Create specific descriptions for different intensity levels of your most problematic modes. What does level 3 Vulnerable Child feel like compared to level 8? How do you behave differently when your Demanding Parent is at level 5 versus level 9?

Include both internal experiences (thoughts, feelings, physical sensations) and external behaviors (what others would observe) in your intensity descriptions.

Identify your typical escalation triggers and patterns. What pushes you from level 3 to level 7? How long does escalation usually take? What factors speed up or slow down the process?

Develop specific coping strategies for different intensity levels. Mild activation might require simple awareness and breathing. Moderate activation might need brief breaks or self-soothing activities. Severe activation might require complete environmental changes or professional support.

Exercise 17: Healthy Adult Mode Strengthening

Building the Adaptive Mode

The Healthy Adult mode represents your wise, balanced, and capable self—the part that can handle life's challenges with flexibility and grace[14]. Unlike other modes that develop as adaptations to childhood difficulties, the Healthy Adult mode represents your authentic, mature self operating from a place of strength and wisdom.

Strengthening this mode involves both developing its capacities and creating conditions that support its emergence. The Healthy Adult mode thrives in environments of safety, authenticity, and meaningful connection, while struggling under conditions of chronic stress, isolation, or emotional chaos.

Case Example: Linda's Leadership Development

Linda, a 41-year-old nonprofit director, worked systematically to strengthen her Healthy Adult mode after recognizing how often her Compliant Surrenderer mode was creating problems at work. Her tendency to avoid conflict and prioritize others' needs over organizational requirements was undermining her effectiveness as a leader.

Linda began by identifying situations where her Healthy Adult mode naturally emerged. These included one-on-one mentoring conversations with junior staff, strategic planning sessions where she could use her analytical skills, and community presentations about her organization's mission. In these contexts, she felt centered, confident, and authentic.

She noticed that her Healthy Adult mode had specific characteristics: clear thinking, emotional balance, genuine confidence (not defensive bravado), natural authority, empathy without enabling, and the ability to set appropriate boundaries. This mode could handle criticism without becoming defensive, express disagreement without attacking, and make difficult decisions with compassion.

Linda practiced strengthening this mode through daily exercises. She began each morning by spending five minutes connecting with her core values and intentions for the day. She practiced expressing her authentic opinions in low-stakes situations before tackling more challenging conversations. She developed a mantra: "I can be kind and strong at the same time."

Over months of practice, Linda's Healthy Adult mode became more accessible during stressful situations. She could disagree with board members without automatically deferring to their opinions. She could address performance problems with staff without either avoiding the issues or becoming overly harsh.

Strengthening Strategies

Identify your Healthy Adult mode's natural strengths and conditions for emergence. When do you feel most balanced, wise, and authentic? What situations bring out your best qualities?

Practice accessing this mode during calm moments before trying to use it during stress. Meditation, journaling, time in nature, or meaningful conversations can help you connect with your Healthy Adult perspective.

Develop specific phrases or mantras that help you access this mode during difficult moments. "I can handle this," "I have everything I need within me," or "I can respond rather than react" are examples.

Set small, achievable goals for using your Healthy Adult mode in challenging situations. Start with low-stakes scenarios and gradually work toward more difficult ones as your confidence builds.

Exercise 18: Child Mode Nurturing Exercises

Caring for Vulnerable and Angry Child Parts

Your Child modes carry the emotional wounds and unmet needs from your earliest years. The Vulnerable Child holds your needs for safety, love, and acceptance, while the Angry Child expresses the rage and protest about unmet needs and poor treatment[15]. Both parts require nurturing attention rather than criticism or suppression.

Child mode nurturing involves providing the comfort, validation, and care that these parts needed but didn't receive during your actual childhood. This isn't regression or self-indulgence—it's therapeutic reparenting that allows wounded parts to heal and integrate.

Case Example: David's Inner Child Healing

David, a 43-year-old engineer, discovered that his Vulnerable Child mode held decades of pain from emotional neglect by parents who were physically present but emotionally unavailable. This part of him still felt like that lonely eight-year-old who tried desperately to get his parents' attention through achievements and good behavior.

David's Vulnerable Child needed validation that his emotional needs were legitimate and important. Through guided exercises, he learned to speak to this part with the warmth and understanding he'd needed as a child. "Of course you wanted love and attention," he would tell his inner child. "Every child deserves to feel valued and cared for. Your needs weren't too much—they were normal and healthy."

David's Angry Child held rage about years of emotional dismissal and criticism. This part was furious about the unfairness of having to earn love through performance while watching other children receive unconditional acceptance. Initially, David tried to suppress this anger, viewing it as inappropriate or dangerous.

Learning to nurture his Angry Child involved validating the legitimate anger while helping this part express it safely. "You have every right to be angry about how you were treated," David acknowledged. "It wasn't fair, and your anger makes complete sense. Let's find healthy ways to express these feelings instead of holding them inside."

David developed specific nurturing practices for each child mode. For his Vulnerable Child, he practiced self-compassion exercises, allowed himself to ask for support from friends, and engaged in comforting activities like warm baths or listening to soothing music. For his Angry Child, he wrote letters expressing his feelings, engaged in vigorous exercise, and practiced assertive communication to express needs directly rather than through passive-aggressive behavior.

46

Nurturing Approaches

Learn the specific language each child mode responds to. The Vulnerable Child often needs gentle, soothing words, while the Angry Child might need validation of its feelings and permission to express them safely.

Provide comfort through multiple senses. Child modes often respond well to physical comfort (soft blankets, warm baths), visual beauty (art, nature), soothing sounds (music, gentle voices), and pleasant scents or tastes.

Create safe spaces for emotional expression. Child modes need permission to feel and express emotions that may have been criticized or suppressed during your actual childhood.

Set appropriate limits with compassion. Child modes sometimes want things that aren't realistic or healthy for adults. The goal is providing emotional nurturing while maintaining adult responsibilities and boundaries.

Exercise 19: Detached Protector Awareness

Recognizing and Working with Emotional Avoidance

The Detached Protector mode serves an important protective function—it shields you from overwhelming emotions and interpersonal pain by creating emotional distance and numbness[16]. While this protection can be lifesaving during trauma or overwhelming stress, chronic activation of this mode cuts you off from both positive and negative emotions, creating a sense of emptiness and disconnection.

Working with the Detached Protector requires understanding its protective function while gradually building tolerance for emotional experience. This mode often developed as a survival strategy during childhood when emotions felt too dangerous or overwhelming to experience fully.

Case Example: Emma's Protective Wall

Emma, a 34-year-old therapist, recognized her Detached Protector mode after noticing how she could discuss her own traumatic childhood with clinical detachment while helping clients process similar experiences with deep empathy. This mode had protected her through years of family chaos and abuse but now interfered with her ability to form intimate relationships.

Emma's Detached Protector had specific triggers: emotional intensity in relationships, conflicts with authority figures, and situations that reminded her of childhood powerlessness. When activated, she would become intellectually engaged but emotionally absent, analyzing situations rather than feeling them.

"It's like watching my life through bulletproof glass," Emma described. "I can see what's happening, but I can't really feel it or connect with it. I'm safe, but I'm also alone."

Working with this mode required Emma to appreciate its protective function while gradually building tolerance for emotional vulnerability. She began by acknowledging the wisdom of this protection: "Thank you for keeping me safe when I was too young to handle all that chaos and pain. You did exactly what I needed you to do."

Emma practiced gradual exposure to emotional experience, starting with low-intensity positive emotions before working toward more vulnerable feelings. She learned to recognize the early signs of detachment and developed strategies for staying emotionally present during difficult conversations.

The key was helping her Detached Protector understand that adult Emma had resources for handling emotions that child Emma hadn't possessed. "I have support now," she would remind this protective part. "I have friends who care about me, professional skills for managing difficult feelings, and the freedom to remove myself from harmful situations. I don't need to shut down completely to stay safe."

Working with Detachment

Recognize the triggers that activate your Detached Protector mode. What situations, emotions, or interpersonal dynamics cause you to become emotionally distant?

Appreciate the protective function this mode has served. Honor its intention to keep you safe rather than criticizing it for creating disconnection.

Practice gradual emotional exposure in safe contexts. Start with mild positive emotions before working toward more vulnerable feelings.

Develop grounding techniques that help you stay present without becoming overwhelmed. These might include breathing exercises, physical sensations, or mindfulness practices.

Build a support network that can help you process emotions safely. The Detached Protector often developed when you had to handle overwhelming experiences alone.

Orchestrating Your Internal World

Mode work transforms your relationship with your internal experience from unconscious reactivity to conscious choice. Instead of being hijacked by different parts of yourself, you become the conductor of your internal orchestra—aware of each instrument's unique voice while creating harmony between them.

This work requires patience and self-compassion. Your modes developed over years or decades and won't change overnight. The goal isn't eliminating difficult modes but creating better relationships between them and strengthening your Healthy Adult mode's capacity to provide wise leadership during challenging times.

The most profound shift often comes from realizing that all your modes make sense given your life experiences. Your Demanding Parent developed to help you achieve and avoid criticism. Your

Vulnerable Child carries your deepest needs for love and connection. Your Detached Protector has kept you safe during overwhelming times. Understanding this logic reduces self-criticism and opens pathways for compassionate internal change.

Key Learning Points

- Schema modes represent different emotional states and behavioral patterns that shift throughout the day
- Mode identification helps recognize which part of yourself is active in any given moment
- Daily tracking reveals patterns in mode activation and provides opportunities for conscious intervention
- Mode dialogues create internal healing through communication between different parts of yourself
- Intensity rating helps calibrate responses and choose appropriate coping strategies
- Strengthening the Healthy Adult mode provides wise leadership for all other parts
- Child modes require nurturing and validation rather than criticism or suppression
- The Detached Protector mode serves important protective functions that should be honored while building emotional tolerance
- Effective mode work balances appreciation for each mode's function with conscious choice about which mode to access in different situations

Chapter 4: Imagery Rescripting Scripts and Exercises

The past lives in your body and nervous system like an underground river, flowing beneath conscious awareness but influencing everything above ground. Traumatic memories don't stay in the past—they become part of your present through the schemas and modes they created. Imagery rescripting offers a powerful method for revisiting these formative experiences and creating new emotional outcomes that can heal old wounds at their source.

This work goes beyond simply talking about the past or gaining intellectual understanding of how childhood experiences shaped your current difficulties. Imagery rescripting engages your visual, emotional, and somatic systems to create new neural pathways that can override old patterns of trauma and neglect[17]. Through guided visualization, you can provide your younger self with the protection, comfort, and validation that was missing during the original experience.

The exercises in this chapter provide systematic approaches to healing traumatic memories while building internal resources for safety and resilience. This isn't about changing what actually happened—it's about changing your internal relationship to those experiences so they no longer control your present-day emotional reactions and behavioral choices.

Exercise 20: Basic Imagery Rescripting Protocol

Step-by-Step Process for Memory Transformation

Imagery rescripting follows a structured protocol that ensures safety while maximizing therapeutic impact. The process involves three main phases: accessing the traumatic memory, rescripting the experience to meet the child's needs, and integrating the new experience into current functioning[18].

Safety and preparation are essential before beginning rescripting work. Clients need adequate emotional regulation skills, a stable therapeutic relationship, and sufficient resources for processing difficult material. Rushing into trauma work without proper preparation can retraumatize rather than heal.

Case Example: Alexandra's Classroom Humiliation

Alexandra, a 29-year-old teacher, worked with a painful memory from third grade that continued to trigger her Defectiveness schema. During a class presentation, she had mispronounced a word, and her teacher had responded with harsh criticism in front of the entire class. "You clearly didn't prepare properly," the teacher had said. "This is what happens when you don't take school seriously."

Eight-year-old Alexandra had felt exposed, ashamed, and convinced that something was fundamentally wrong with her. The experience became a foundational memory for beliefs about her inadequacy and the danger of making mistakes in public.

The rescripting process began with Alexandra connecting to the memory while maintaining her adult perspective. "I can see myself as that eight-year-old girl," she described. "I'm wearing my favorite purple dress, and I'm so excited to share my report about dolphins. Then I mispronounce 'echolocation,' and everything changes."

In the original memory, young Alexandra had stood frozen while classmates laughed and the teacher continued criticizing. Adult Alexandra entered the image to provide protection and comfort. "I walk into that classroom and I can see how small and scared she looks," Alexandra narrated. "I go to her and put my arm around her shoulders."

The rescripting involved several interventions. Adult Alexandra confronted the teacher: "That's not how you speak to a child who's trying her best. She's eight years old and she's nervous. Your job is to encourage her, not humiliate her." She comforted young Alexandra: "You did nothing wrong. That word is hard to pronounce, and you prepared really well for this presentation. I'm proud of you for trying."

The rescripted version concluded with young Alexandra receiving the support she needed—encouragement from her adult self, apologies from the teacher, and validation from classmates who told her they enjoyed learning about dolphins. The new memory ended with young Alexandra feeling proud of her effort rather than ashamed of her mistake.

Implementation Guidelines

Begin with careful memory selection. Start with moderately distressing memories rather than the most traumatic ones. Early rescripting work builds skills and confidence for tackling more difficult material later.

Create detailed sensory descriptions of the original memory. What did you see, hear, smell, or physically feel? Rich sensory details help access the emotional content of the memory more fully.

Enter the image as your current adult self rather than trying to change the child's behavior. The adult you has resources, knowledge, and power that the child didn't possess.

Focus on meeting the child's emotional needs rather than just stopping the abuse or neglect. What did your younger self need in that moment? Comfort? Protection? Validation? Understanding?

End rescripting sessions with positive, nurturing scenes. The child should feel safe, comforted, and valued by the end of the process.

Exercise 21: Safe Place Visualization

Creating a Protective Internal Environment

Safe place visualization creates an internal sanctuary that you can access during difficult times or when processing traumatic material. This imagined place serves as a resource for self-soothing and emotional regulation, providing a sense of safety that may have been missing during your childhood experiences.

The safe place isn't just a pleasant fantasy—it's a carefully constructed psychological resource that engages your nervous system's capacity for calming and self-regulation. Regular practice with safe place imagery strengthens your ability to access calm states even during stress or trauma processing.

Case Example: Marcus's Mountain Retreat

Marcus, a 36-year-old paramedic, created a safe place visualization to help manage PTSD symptoms from both childhood abuse and work-related trauma. His safe place was a cabin in the mountains, surrounded by tall pine trees and situated next to a clear, flowing stream.

"I can hear the water moving over the rocks," Marcus described. "It's a constant, peaceful sound that drowns out any other noise. The air smells like pine and fresh water. There's a comfortable chair on the porch where I can sit and watch the trees sway in the breeze."

The cabin had specific protective features that addressed Marcus's trauma history. The doors had strong locks that only he controlled. The windows provided clear views in all directions so he could see anyone approaching. Inside, there was a cozy fireplace, soft blankets, and a well-stocked kitchen—symbols of warmth, comfort, and nourishment.

Marcus practiced visiting his safe place daily, spending 10-15 minutes in visualization to strengthen his ability to access this resource. During particularly difficult shifts at work or when processing traumatic memories in therapy, he could briefly connect with his mountain retreat to regulate his nervous system and restore a sense of safety.

The safe place also became a launching point for other imagery work. Before rescripting traumatic memories, Marcus would start in his mountain cabin, gathering strength and resources before entering more difficult material. This approach helped him maintain connection to safety even while processing painful experiences.

Safe Place Construction

Choose a location that feels naturally peaceful and secure to you. This might be a real place you've visited, a combination of several places, or a completely imagined location.

Include multiple sensory details to make the experience vivid and engaging. What do you see, hear, smell, feel, or taste in your safe place? Rich sensory details enhance the calming effect.

Add protective elements that address your specific safety concerns. These might include locks, barriers, protective animals, or supernatural elements that ensure your complete security.

Include nurturing resources like comfortable furniture, food, warmth, or entertainment. Your safe place should meet both safety and comfort needs.

Practice accessing your safe place regularly when you're already calm. This strengthens the neural pathways associated with the visualization, making it more accessible during stress.

Exercise 22: Childhood Rescue Scenarios

Adult Self Protecting the Child Self

Childhood rescue scenarios involve your adult self entering traumatic childhood situations to provide protection, comfort, and advocacy that was missing during the original experience. This work directly addresses helplessness and abandonment feelings that often form the core of schema development.

Rescue scenarios tap into your adult capacities for strength, wisdom, and resources while healing the wounded child parts that still carry trauma. The adult you can do things that the child couldn't—set boundaries, call for help, remove yourself from danger, or confront abusive adults.

Case Example: Jennifer's Playground Protection

Jennifer, a 31-year-old social worker, used rescue scenarios to heal memories of severe bullying during elementary school. One particularly painful memory involved being surrounded by a group of older children who pushed her down, took her lunch money, and called her ugly names while other children watched without intervening.

In the original memory, six-year-old Jennifer felt completely helpless and alone. She couldn't defend herself against larger children, and no adults were present to help. The experience created beliefs about her powerlessness and the unreliability of others for support.

The rescue scenario began with adult Jennifer arriving at the playground just as the bullying started. "I can see those kids surrounding my younger self," Jennifer narrated. "She looks so small and scared. I walk over with complete confidence—I'm bigger than all of them, and I have adult authority."

Adult Jennifer confronted the bullies directly: "Stop right now. This is completely unacceptable behavior, and it ends immediately." She helped young Jennifer stand up and checked to make sure she wasn't hurt. "You're safe now," she told her younger self. "I'm here, and I won't let anyone hurt you."

The scenario included consequences for the bullies—adult Jennifer marched them to the principal's office and ensured they faced appropriate discipline. She also advocated for young Jennifer, explaining to school staff how the bullying was affecting her and demanding better supervision during recess.

The rescue concluded with adult Jennifer taking young Jennifer somewhere safe and comforting—her grandmother's house, where they had warm cookies and talked about the incident. Young Jennifer learned that she deserved protection, that adults could be trusted to help, and that she wasn't powerless against those who wanted to hurt her.

Rescue Scenario Guidelines

Enter scenarios with your full adult strength, wisdom, and resources. You're not trying to make the child braver or stronger—you're providing external protection and support.

Address both immediate safety and longer-term consequences. Stop the abuse or neglect, but also ensure the child receives ongoing protection and care.

Include other supportive adults when helpful. Sometimes rescue scenarios benefit from police, teachers, relatives, or other protective figures joining your efforts.

Focus on the child's emotional needs as well as physical safety. Provide comfort, validation, and reassurance that addresses the psychological impact of the trauma.

End scenarios with the child feeling genuinely safe and cared for. The goal is creating new emotional experiences, not just stopping the traumatic events.

Exercise 23: Parental Re-scripting Exercise

Imagining Healthier Parental Responses

Parental re-scripting involves reimagining how your parents or caregivers might have responded differently to your childhood needs and behaviors. This work addresses the internalized critical or neglectful parent voices that continue to shape your self-talk and self-treatment as an adult.

This exercise isn't about excusing harmful parental behavior or pretending abuse didn't happen. It's about providing your younger self with examples of healthy parental responses that can serve as models for how you treat yourself and others now.

Case Example: Robert's Emotional Validation

Robert, a 38-year-old accountant, worked with memories of his father's emotional dismissal during childhood. Whenever young Robert expressed fear, sadness, or vulnerability, his father would respond with phrases like "Stop being a baby," "Big boys don't cry," or "You're too sensitive."

One specific memory involved eight-year-old Robert crying after his pet hamster died. His father had become angry about the tears, telling Robert that "It's just an animal" and that he needed to "toughen up" if he wanted to be successful in life. Young Robert had learned to suppress his emotions and developed beliefs about emotional expression being weakness.

The re-scripting exercise involved imagining how a healthy father might have responded to his grief. In the new version, Robert's father sits down beside his crying son and asks what's wrong. When Robert explains about his hamster, the re-scripted father responds with empathy: "I'm so sorry about your hamster. You really loved him, didn't you? It's completely normal to feel sad when someone we care about dies."

The healthy father validates Robert's emotions: "Caring about others and feeling sad when we lose them shows that you have a good heart. Those are wonderful qualities, not weaknesses." He offers comfort: "Would you like to have a little funeral for your hamster? We could bury him in the backyard and say some nice things about how much joy he brought you."

The re-scripted interaction ends with young Robert feeling understood and supported rather than ashamed and isolated. The healthy father models emotional intelligence and shows Robert that feelings are normal and manageable rather than dangerous or shameful.

Through repeated practice with parental re-scripting, Robert began internalizing these healthier parental voices. When he felt overwhelmed or emotional as an adult, he could access the caring, wise parent from his re-scripted memories rather than the critical, dismissive voice from his actual childhood.

Re-scripting Approaches

Focus on one parent or caregiver at a time to avoid confusion or overwhelm. You can work with both parents separately in different exercises.

Identify specific qualities you needed from your parents—empathy, validation, protection, guidance, encouragement, or unconditional love. Let these needs guide how you re-script their responses.

Keep parental responses realistic and believable. The goal isn't creating perfect fantasy parents but imaging how emotionally healthy parents might have responded.

Include both emotional responses (validation, comfort) and practical actions (protection, advocacy, teaching) in your re-scripted interactions.

Practice accessing these healthier parental voices during current difficulties. The internalized healthy parent can provide ongoing support and guidance throughout your adult life.

Exercise 24: Future Self Imagery

Connecting with a Healed Version of Oneself

Future self imagery involves connecting with a version of yourself that has healed from current struggles and achieved greater emotional health and life satisfaction. This exercise provides hope, motivation, and practical guidance by accessing the wisdom of your potential future self.

The future self represents not a perfect person without problems, but someone who has learned to handle life's challenges with greater skill, self-compassion, and resilience. This version of you has done the healing work and can offer encouragement and advice for your current journey.

Case Example: Sarah's Wise Future Self

Sarah, a 27-year-old graduate student struggling with anxiety and self-doubt, connected with her future self at age 45. In the imagery, she met a version of herself who was calm, confident, and genuinely happy. This future Sarah worked as a professor, had a loving relationship, and maintained close friendships—all things that current Sarah worried she might never achieve.

"She looks peaceful," Sarah described. "Not like she never has problems, but like she knows how to handle them. There's this quiet confidence about her that I don't have yet. She seems genuinely comfortable in her own skin."

Future Sarah offered encouragement about current struggles: "I know everything feels overwhelming right now, and you're scared that you'll never feel better. But I'm here to tell you that you will. The anxiety doesn't last forever, and the work you're doing now—the therapy, the self-reflection, the courage to face your fears—it all pays off."

She provided practical advice: "Stop trying to be perfect. That's what's making you so miserable. You're already good enough, and you always have been. Start saying no to things that drain you and yes to things that feed your soul. Trust your instincts—they're better than you think."

Future Sarah also shared specific strategies that had helped: "Meditation really does work, even though it feels impossible at first. Keep practicing. And that therapist you're working with? Trust her process. She knows what she's doing. The scariest work turns out to be the most healing."

60

The imagery session ended with future Sarah giving current Sarah a warm hug and a reminder: "You're braver than you know, and you're worthy of all the good things coming your way. I'm proud of you for not giving up."

Future Self Connection

Choose an age that represents a significantly healed version of yourself—usually 10-20 years in the future. This gives enough time for meaningful growth and change.

Create a detailed image of your future self. What do they look like? How do they carry themselves? What's different about their energy or presence?

Focus on emotional and psychological qualities rather than just external achievements. How does your future self handle stress, relationships, and challenges?

Ask your future self specific questions about current struggles. What advice would they give? What do they wish current you knew?

End sessions with receiving some form of gift, blessing, or encouragement from your future self. This could be words of wisdom, an object that represents their support, or simply their confidence in your ability to heal and grow.

Exercise 25: Resource Installation

Building Internal Strength and Resilience

Resource installation involves using imagery to build internal capacities for strength, wisdom, comfort, and resilience. Rather than just processing traumatic memories, this work actively constructs positive resources that can support you during difficult times.

These resources might include protective figures, symbols of strength, sources of wisdom, or connections to larger meaning and purpose.

The goal is creating internal assets that are always available, regardless of external circumstances.

Case Example: Michael's Protective Council

Michael, a 41-year-old manager who struggled with feelings of inadequacy and vulnerability, created an internal council of protective and wise figures through resource installation work. His council included his deceased grandfather (who represented unconditional love), a favorite teacher (who embodied encouragement and belief in his potential), and an imagined wise warrior (who provided strength and courage).

"I can see them sitting around a table in a comfortable room," Michael described. "My grandfather has that gentle smile he always had, Mrs. Johnson looks at me with those encouraging eyes, and the warrior sits quietly but I can feel his strength and protection."

Michael's grandfather offered comfort during times of self-doubt: "You are deeply loved just as you are. Nothing you do or don't do changes that. You don't have to earn love—it's already yours."

His teacher provided encouragement during challenges: "I always saw your potential, even when you couldn't see it yourself. You have talents and abilities that the world needs. Don't let fear stop you from sharing your gifts."

The wise warrior offered strength during confrontations or difficult decisions: "You have more courage than you realize. Stand tall, speak your truth, and trust your inner wisdom. I am here to lend you strength whenever you need it."

Michael practiced accessing his council regularly, especially before difficult conversations or challenging situations. Over time, these resource figures became internalized sources of support that he could access even without formal imagery practice.

Installation Techniques

Choose resource figures that represent qualities you need to develop or strengthen. These might be real people, fictional characters, spiritual figures, or archetypal representations.

Create detailed visualizations of each resource, including their appearance, energy, and the specific qualities they embody.

Develop specific phrases or messages that each resource figure offers. What would they say to comfort, encourage, or strengthen you?

Practice accessing these resources during calm times before trying to use them during stress or difficulty.

Allow your resource council to evolve over time. New figures might emerge as you grow and heal, while others might recede as their particular gifts become internalized.

Exercise 26: Somatic Imagery Integration

Connecting Body Sensations with Healing Images

Trauma and schema formation involve both psychological and physical dimensions. Somatic imagery integration works with the body's wisdom and healing capacity by connecting physical sensations with healing imagery. This approach recognizes that lasting change often requires engagement with the nervous system and somatic experience.

The body holds memories and patterns that purely cognitive approaches might miss. By including somatic awareness in imagery work, you can address trauma at the cellular level where it's often stored.

Case Example: Lisa's Heart Healing

Lisa, a 35-year-old nurse, worked with chronic chest tightness and heart palpitations that worscned during stress or interpersonal conflict. Medical testing had ruled out physical causes, suggesting these symptoms were related to her history of emotional abuse and rejection.

During somatic imagery work, Lisa connected with her heart area and noticed sensations of constriction, heaviness, and rapid beating. "It feels like my heart is in a cage," she described. "It's trying to beat normally, but it can't expand fully."

The imagery work involved visualizing the cage around her heart—made of dark, heavy metal with sharp edges. Lisa explored this image with curiosity: "What is this cage protecting me from? What would happen if it opened?"

She realized the cage represented protection against further heartbreak and rejection. Young Lisa had developed this armor after repeated experiences of emotional abandonment and criticism. The cage protected her heart but also prevented her from fully receiving love and connection.

The healing imagery involved gradually opening the cage while maintaining safety. Lisa visualized warm, golden light flowing into her heart area, dissolving the metal bars slowly and gently. "I can keep the protection I need while allowing my heart to expand and breathe," she told herself.

The physical sensations shifted during the imagery—the tightness began releasing, her breathing deepened, and the heart palpitations settled into a steady, strong rhythm. Lisa ended the session by placing both hands on her heart and sending herself the love and acceptance her heart had been craving.

Regular practice with this somatic imagery helped Lisa's chronic chest symptoms improve significantly. More importantly, she became more open to emotional intimacy and connection in her relationships.

Somatic Integration Methods

Begin with body awareness exercises to identify areas of tension, numbness, or discomfort that might hold trauma or emotional patterns.

Use imagery to explore physical sensations with curiosity rather than judgment. What does this tension look like? What color or texture does it have? What might it be protecting?

Include movement, breathing, or sound in your imagery work when helpful. Sometimes the body needs to express or release energy during healing processes.

Work slowly and gently with somatic material. The body's wisdom includes protective mechanisms that shouldn't be forced or rushed.

End somatic imagery sessions by sending appreciation and care to your body for its wisdom and resilience throughout difficult experiences.

Healing Through Imagined Experience

Imagery rescripting represents one of the most powerful tools available for healing trauma and changing deep psychological patterns. By engaging visual, emotional, and somatic systems simultaneously, this work creates new neural pathways that can override old patterns of fear, shame, and helplessness.

The exercises in this chapter provide systematic approaches to different aspects of imagery healing—from basic rescripting protocols to resource installation and somatic integration. Each approach offers unique benefits while contributing to overall emotional healing and resilience building.

Success with imagery work requires patience, practice, and often professional guidance, especially when working with severe trauma. However, the potential for healing is enormous. Unlike purely cognitive approaches that work with thoughts and beliefs, imagery work can create new emotional experiences that heal wounds at their source.

The goal isn't erasing the past or pretending difficult experiences didn't happen. Instead, imagery rescripting changes your internal relationship to those experiences, reducing their power to control your present-day emotional reactions and behavioral choices. Through this work, you can become the author of your own healing story.

Core Principles for Practice

- Imagery rescripting engages multiple systems (visual, emotional, somatic) to create comprehensive healing experiences
- Safety and emotional regulation skills are essential prerequisites for trauma processing work
- The adult self provides resources and protection that weren't available during original traumatic experiences
- Safe place visualization creates internal sanctuaries for self-regulation and emotional stability
- Rescue scenarios address helplessness and abandonment through adult intervention and protection
- Parental re-scripting provides models of healthy responses that can be internalized for ongoing self-care
- Future self imagery offers hope, motivation, and practical wisdom for current healing work
- Resource installation builds positive internal assets for strength, comfort, and resilience
- Somatic integration addresses trauma at the nervous system level where it's often stored

Chapter 5: Chair Work and Dialogue Techniques

Internal conflicts often feel like having multiple people arguing inside your head, each with their own agenda and volume control. Chair work makes these internal voices literal by giving them actual seats at the table—or rather, actual chairs in the therapy room. This deceptively simple technique transforms abstract psychological concepts into concrete, workable conversations between different parts of yourself.

The power of chair work lies in its ability to externalize what usually happens internally and unconsciously. Instead of being overwhelmed by competing thoughts and feelings, you can sit in one chair and speak as your critical voice, then move to another chair and respond as your vulnerable self. This physical movement engages your body and nervous system in ways that purely cognitive work cannot match[19].

Chair work creates space for parts of yourself that rarely get heard in daily life. Your inner critic might dominate most conversations, but in chair work, your wise adult self gets equal time and positioning. The technique doesn't try to eliminate difficult parts—it helps them communicate more effectively and find better ways to meet their underlying needs.

Exercise 27: Basic Two-Chair Setup

Fundamental Chair Work Structure

The basic two-chair setup provides the foundation for all chair work interventions. This technique involves placing two chairs facing each other and using them to represent different aspects of yourself, other people, or conflicting perspectives. The physical act of moving between chairs helps access different emotional states and viewpoints more fully than mental imagination alone.

Proper setup and facilitation make the difference between powerful therapeutic work and awkward role-playing. The chairs should be positioned close enough for intimate conversation but far enough apart to feel like distinct spaces. The facilitator's role involves guiding transitions, encouraging full expression, and helping maintain safety throughout the process.

Case Example: Maria's Perfectionist Struggle

Maria, a 34-year-old architect, used basic two-chair work to address the internal battle between her perfectionist standards and her need for self-acceptance. One chair represented her Demanding Parent mode—the harsh, critical voice that insisted everything must be flawless. The other chair held her Vulnerable Child mode—the part that felt exhausted and defeated by impossible standards.

Sitting in the Demanding Parent chair, Maria's voice became sharp and urgent: "You can't submit that design yet. Look at all those flaws! The proportions are slightly off in the third section, and the materials list isn't completely optimized. If you turn this in now, everyone will see that you're not as good as they thought. You'll lose respect and probably get fired."

Moving to the Vulnerable Child chair, Maria's posture changed—her shoulders slumped, her voice became smaller: "I'm so tired of never being good enough. I've been working on this project for weeks, and no matter what I do, you find something wrong with it. I just want to feel proud of my work for once. I want to go home and see my family instead of staying here until midnight again."

The dialogue continued with each part expressing their fears and needs. The Demanding Parent revealed its terror of failure and rejection: "I'm trying to protect you from humiliation. I've seen what happens to people who aren't careful enough—they get criticized, passed over, forgotten." The Vulnerable Child expressed its need for acceptance and rest: "I need to know that I'm okay even when my work isn't perfect. I need to feel valued for who I am, not just what I produce."

Through multiple sessions of chair work, Maria began developing a third voice—her Healthy Adult mode—that could appreciate both parts' concerns while finding a middle path. This adult voice could acknowledge the value of high standards while recognizing when perfectionism became self-destructive.

Setup and Facilitation Guidelines

Position chairs at a comfortable conversational distance—typically 3-4 feet apart. The chairs should be of equal height and comfort to avoid creating power dynamics through furniture choices.

Begin with clear instructions about the process. Explain that the person will be speaking from different parts of themselves and that moving between chairs helps access these different perspectives.

Encourage full expression in each chair before prompting transitions. Let each voice say everything it needs to say before moving to the other perspective.

Use physical cues to support transitions. "Now move to the other chair and respond as your wise adult self" creates clearer boundaries than purely verbal instructions.

Maintain safety by monitoring emotional intensity and providing grounding if needed. Chair work can activate powerful emotions that require careful containment.

Exercise 28: Schema vs. Healthy Adult Dialogue

Conversations Between Maladaptive and Adaptive Parts

Schema versus Healthy Adult dialogues create structured conversations between schema-driven parts and your wise, balanced adult self. This technique helps you recognize how schemas operate while strengthening your capacity to respond from a healthier perspective. The schema voice expresses fears, demands, and automatic reactions, while the Healthy Adult provides rational alternatives and emotional support.

These dialogues serve multiple purposes: they externalize schema patterns for clearer recognition, provide practice responding to schema activation, and strengthen the Healthy Adult mode through repeated use. Over time, these external conversations become internalized as healthier self-talk patterns.

Case Example: David's Abandonment Recovery

David, a 31-year-old teacher, struggled with an Abandonment schema that created intense anxiety in relationships. His schema voice would become activated whenever his girlfriend seemed distant or busy, flooding him with fears of rejection and demands for constant reassurance.

In the schema chair, David's voice became anxious and demanding: "She didn't text back for three hours. That means she's losing interest. You need to call her right now and find out what's wrong. Maybe send flowers or plan something special to win her back. You can't just ignore this—she's definitely pulling away."

Moving to the Healthy Adult chair, David's posture straightened and his voice became calmer: "I understand you're scared because Sarah seemed quiet during dinner last night. But three hours isn't a long time to wait for a text. She mentioned having a big presentation today, so she's probably focused on work. Our relationship has been solid for months—one quiet evening doesn't mean it's ending."

The schema voice responded with more urgency: "But what if you're wrong? What if she's already checked out emotionally and you're just fooling yourself? You should at least check her social media to see if she's posting normally. Or maybe text her something casual to test her response."

The Healthy Adult chair offered perspective and alternatives: "Even if Sarah is having doubts about our relationship, anxious texting and checking up on her will push her away rather than bring her closer.

70

The best thing I can do is be my authentic self and trust that our connection is strong enough to handle normal relationship fluctuations. If she needs space, I can give it to her while maintaining my own emotional stability."

Through repeated practice with these dialogues, David learned to recognize his schema voice earlier and access his Healthy Adult response more quickly. The conversations became shorter and more automatic as his healthy patterns strengthened.

Dialogue Implementation

Clearly identify which schema will sit in the first chair before beginning the conversation. Name it specifically—"This chair is for your Abandonment schema" rather than just "your fears."

Encourage the schema voice to express its full concerns without immediate challenge or correction. Schemas need to feel heard before they'll consider alternative perspectives.

Help the Healthy Adult voice respond with both empathy and alternative viewpoints. "I understand why you're scared, and here's another way to look at this situation."

Practice these dialogues regularly, not just during crisis moments. Building the Healthy Adult voice requires consistent exercise, like strengthening a muscle.

Allow the conversations to be messy and repetitive. Schemas don't change quickly, and the Healthy Adult voice needs time to develop convincing alternatives.

Exercise 29: Empty Chair for Deceased/Absent Figures

Resolving Unfinished Business

The empty chair technique for deceased or absent figures provides opportunities to complete conversations that were never finished, express feelings that were never shared, and gain closure on relationships that ended without resolution. This work doesn't require the other person's presence or cooperation—it focuses on your own healing and emotional completion[20].

Unfinished business often involves things we wish we had said, questions we never asked, or emotions we never expressed. These unexpressed communications can create ongoing psychological tension that affects current relationships and self-concept. Chair work provides a safe space to finally have these conversations.

Case Example: Jennifer's Father Dialogue

Jennifer, a 38-year-old social worker, used empty chair work to address unfinished business with her father, who had died suddenly when she was 16. Their relationship had been tense during her adolescence, with frequent conflicts about her choices and behavior. His death had left her carrying guilt, anger, and unexpressed love.

Sitting across from the empty chair representing her father, Jennifer began tentatively: "I've been angry at you for fifteen years, but I've also missed you every single day. I never got to tell you that I understood why you were so strict with me. You were worried about me making mistakes that would hurt my future."

As the conversation continued, Jennifer's emotions intensified: "But you never told me you loved me, Dad. You criticized everything I did, and I started believing that I wasn't good enough for anyone. I've spent my whole adult life trying to prove I'm worthy of love, and I'm exhausted."

Speaking as her father, Jennifer accessed a more understanding perspective: "I did love you, sweetheart. I was just scared of showing too much emotion because that's not how I was raised. When I criticized you, I was trying to prepare you for a world that would be even harsher. I wanted you to be strong enough to handle anything."

The dialogue allowed Jennifer to express forgiveness: "I forgive you for not knowing how to show love in ways I could understand. You

72

did the best you could with what you learned from your own parents."
She also received the validation she'd needed: "I wish I had told you
more often how proud I was of your compassion and intelligence.
You were never not good enough—you were exactly the daughter I
hoped for."

The conversation concluded with Jennifer feeling lighter and more
complete. She hadn't changed what happened between them, but she'd
changed her relationship to those experiences.

Working with Absent Figures

Begin by establishing a clear sense of the other person's presence in
the empty chair. What would they look like? How would they sit?
What would their energy feel like?

Start with whatever feelings are most present—anger, sadness, love,
confusion. There's no "right" way to begin these conversations.

Include both expressing your feelings and speaking as the other
person. Try to access their perspective as you understand it, not just
your wishes for what they might say.

Allow for multiple sessions if needed. Complex relationships often
require several conversations to reach completion.

End with some form of closure—forgiveness, acceptance, or simply
acknowledgment of what was and wasn't possible in that relationship.

Exercise 30: Inner Critic Confrontation

Challenging Self-Critical Voices

The inner critic represents one of the most common and damaging
voices in human psychology—the internal narrator that focuses
relentlessly on mistakes, inadequacies, and potential failures. Inner
critic confrontation uses chair work to externalize this voice and
develop stronger responses to its attacks. This technique helps you

recognize the critic's patterns, understand its origins, and build immunity to its harmful messages.

Most people experience their inner critic as their own voice, making it difficult to challenge or question. Chair work creates distance by putting the critic in a separate chair, allowing you to see its patterns more objectively and respond from a stronger position.

Case Example: Robert's Harsh Judge

Robert, a 29-year-old engineer, struggled with a particularly vicious inner critic that attacked every decision he made and every mistake he noticed. The voice had become so automatic that Robert often didn't realize how brutally he was treating himself internally.

In the critic chair, Robert's voice became harsh and absolute: "You're such an idiot for making that calculation error in the meeting today. Everyone probably thinks you're incompetent now. You should have caught that mistake—any decent engineer would have. You're probably going to get fired, and you'll deserve it for being so careless."

Moving to his adult self chair, Robert initially felt overwhelmed by the critic's intensity: "I... I don't know how to respond to that. Maybe you're right. Maybe I really am incompetent."

With practice, Robert learned to challenge the critic more effectively: "Wait a minute. One calculation error doesn't make me incompetent. I've successfully completed dozens of projects, and my evaluations have always been positive. Everyone makes mistakes sometimes— that's how we learn and improve. The error was caught and corrected, so no real harm was done."

The critic responded with more attacks: "You're just making excuses. Successful people don't make careless mistakes. You should be perfect if you want to get anywhere in this field."

Robert's adult voice grew stronger: "That's completely unrealistic. No one is perfect, and expecting perfection from myself just creates anxiety that actually makes mistakes more likely. I'm a competent engineer who occasionally makes errors, just like every other human being in any profession."

Through repeated confrontations, Robert learned to recognize his critic's voice earlier and respond with more balanced self-talk. The critic didn't disappear, but it lost much of its power to create shame and self-doubt.

Confrontation Strategies

Identify the specific language and tone your inner critic uses. Does it use "you" statements, absolutes like "always" and "never," or comparisons to others?

Help your adult voice respond with both challenge and self-compassion. "That's not accurate, and even if it were, I still deserve kindness."

Question the critic's evidence and logic. "What proof do you have for that statement? Are you applying realistic standards?"

Explore the critic's origins and intentions. Often, harsh self-criticism developed as protection against external criticism or rejection.

Practice the confrontation regularly, not just during crisis moments. Building resistance to critical voices requires consistent practice.

Exercise 31: Parent-Child Chair Work

Processing Childhood Relationships

Parent-child chair work creates opportunities to process unresolved feelings about childhood relationships, express emotions that were suppressed during development, and develop more balanced perspectives on parental figures. This technique recognizes that our relationships with parents continue to influence us throughout adulthood, often in ways we don't fully recognize.

The work involves both expressing feelings to parents and accessing more adult perspectives on their behavior. The goal isn't excusing harmful parental actions but developing understanding that reduces the emotional charge of childhood experiences.

Case Example: Susan's Mother Conversation

Susan, a 42-year-old therapist, used parent-child chair work to process her relationship with a mother who had been emotionally cold and critical throughout Susan's childhood. Susan had developed beliefs about being unlovable and burdensome that continued to affect her adult relationships.

Speaking to her mother's chair, Susan expressed decades of hurt: "You never seemed happy to see me. When I came home from school excited about something, you would point out my messy hair or ask why I hadn't finished my chores. I needed you to be proud of me, to light up when I walked in the room, but you always seemed irritated by my presence."

Accessing her child voice, Susan continued: "I tried so hard to be good enough for you. I got straight A's, cleaned my room perfectly, never asked for anything I didn't absolutely need. But nothing I did ever seemed to make you happy. I started believing that something was wrong with me, that I was just naturally disappointing to people."

Speaking as her mother, Susan accessed a more complex perspective: "I was overwhelmed and depressed, though I didn't understand that at the time. Your father worked long hours, I had three children and no help, and I felt like I was drowning most days. When I criticized you, I thought I was teaching you to be better prepared for life's challenges."

The mother voice continued: "I didn't know how to express love and pride because my own mother never did that for me. I was proud of you, but I was afraid that if I praised you too much, you'd become spoiled or lazy. I thought criticism would motivate you to achieve more."

76

This conversation helped Susan understand her mother's limitations without excusing the harm caused: "I can see that you were struggling and did the best you could with the tools you had. But the criticism and emotional distance damaged my self-worth in ways I'm still healing from. I needed more warmth and acceptance than you were able to give."

Parent Work Guidelines

Begin with expressing your authentic feelings—hurt, anger, disappointment, or love. Don't censor emotions to protect the parent's feelings.

Include both child and adult perspectives. Your inner child needs to express hurt, while your adult self can offer more complex understanding.

Try to access your parent's perspective without excusing harmful behavior. Understanding doesn't require agreement or absolution.

Focus on your own healing rather than changing or fixing the parental relationship. This work is about your internal relationship to these experiences.

Allow for grief about what was and wasn't possible in these relationships. Some losses require mourning before healing can occur.

Exercise 32: Mode-to-Mode Conversations

Dialogue Between Different Schema Modes

Mode-to-mode conversations create structured dialogues between different parts of your personality, allowing each mode to express its needs and perspectives while working toward better internal cooperation. These conversations help modes understand each other rather than working at cross-purposes or switching rapidly without communication.

Unlike traditional chair work that focuses on specific conflicts, mode conversations involve multiple aspects of your personality learning to collaborate more effectively. The goal is internal harmony rather than dominance by any single mode.

Case Example: Michael's Internal Team Meeting

Michael, a 35-year-old manager, struggled with rapid mode switching that left him feeling chaotic and unpredictable. His Vulnerable Child mode would become activated by criticism, his Demanding Parent would try to regain control through perfectionism, and his Detached Protector would shut down emotionally when the pressure became too intense.

Using three chairs, Michael facilitated a conversation between these modes. His Vulnerable Child spoke first: "I'm tired of being attacked all the time. Every time someone criticizes our work, I feel like that scared little boy who could never do anything right. I just want to feel safe and accepted, but you two always take over before I can even process what's happening."

The Demanding Parent responded: "I'm trying to protect you from more criticism by making sure everything we do is perfect. If I don't push us to work harder and do better, people will see that we're not good enough, and then we'll really be in trouble. The criticism would get worse, not better."

The Detached Protector added: "And when you two get into these battles, the emotional intensity becomes overwhelming. I shut everything down so we can function without falling apart completely. I'm trying to protect us from being destroyed by all these feelings."

Through guided conversation, the modes began understanding each other's intentions: "We're all trying to protect Michael, but we're working against each other instead of together. What if we could find ways to cooperate?"

The Vulnerable Child expressed its needs: "I need to feel heard when I'm scared, not immediately pushed aside or shut down." The

Demanding Parent adjusted its approach: "I could focus on realistic standards instead of perfectionism, and check with the Vulnerable Child before pushing too hard." The Detached Protector offered compromise: "I could provide calm and stability without completely shutting down emotional connection."

Over time, these internal conversations became more automatic, helping Michael's modes coordinate better during stressful situations.

Mode Conversation Structure

Identify the primary modes that need better communication. Start with two or three modes rather than trying to include all possible parts.

Give each mode dedicated time to express its perspective, needs, and concerns without interruption from other modes.

Help modes understand each other's positive intentions. Most modes developed to serve protective or adaptive functions.

Work toward collaborative solutions that meet everyone's needs rather than having one mode dominate others.

Practice these conversations regularly to strengthen internal communication and cooperation.

Exercise 33: Relationship Conflict Resolution

Practicing Difficult Conversations

Chair work provides a safe laboratory for practicing difficult conversations before having them in real relationships. This technique allows you to explore different approaches, anticipate the other person's responses, and develop confidence for challenging interactions. The practice can reveal your assumptions, fears, and habitual patterns while building skills for more effective communication.

Relationship conflict resolution through chair work helps separate your projections and fears from the actual relationship dynamics. Often, our anticipation of others' responses is colored by past experiences or schema patterns rather than current realities.

Case Example: Linda's Boss Confrontation

Linda, a 33-year-old marketing manager, needed to address a problematic pattern with her boss, who consistently took credit for Linda's ideas in meetings. Linda's Submissive schema made it difficult for her to assert herself directly, while her Angry Child wanted to explode with accusations and demands.

In chair work preparation, Linda first spoke from her Angry Child mode: "You keep stealing my ideas and presenting them as your own! I'm tired of watching you get promoted while I do all the work. It's not fair, and I'm not going to put up with it anymore. Either give me credit or I'm going to report you to HR."

Then Linda accessed her boss's potential perspective: "I'm not stealing your ideas—I'm managing our team's output and presenting it at the appropriate level. You're junior staff, so naturally the ideas get filtered through management before reaching executives. If you want more recognition, you need to develop better presentation skills and understand organizational hierarchy."

Linda tried a more balanced approach from her Healthy Adult mode: "I've noticed that several ideas I've proposed in our team meetings have been presented to upper management without attribution to me. I understand that you need to synthesize team input, but I'd appreciate being acknowledged for my specific contributions, especially on the Johnson campaign strategy that was originally my concept."

The practice revealed Linda's fears: "What if she gets angry and retaliates? What if she says the ideas weren't really mine? What if I sound whiny or entitled?" Working through these fears helped Linda develop responses and build confidence for the actual conversation.

After several practice sessions, Linda approached her boss with clear, professional language and realistic expectations. The conversation went better than anticipated, resulting in an agreement about attribution and Linda's increased involvement in client presentations.

Conflict Resolution Practice

Choose specific conversations that you need to have rather than practicing general confrontation skills. Concrete scenarios produce more useful practice.

Explore your worst-case scenario fears first. What's the absolute worst thing that could happen? How would you handle that outcome?

Practice multiple approaches—from your various modes and from different emotional states. This builds flexibility for responding to unexpected reactions.

Include listening and empathy in your practice, not just expressing your perspective. Effective conversations require understanding the other person's viewpoint.

Focus on your goals for the conversation. What outcome do you want, and what would represent success even if you don't get everything you hope for?

Breaking Through Internal Barriers

Chair work transforms abstract psychological concepts into concrete, workable experiences. Instead of talking about your inner critic, you can sit across from it and have a real conversation. Instead of feeling overwhelmed by conflicting emotions, you can give each feeling its own chair and time to speak.

The power of these techniques lies in their ability to create new experiences rather than just new understanding. Your nervous system learns differently through embodied practice than through cognitive discussion alone. Chair work engages your whole being in the healing process.

These exercises provide tools for ongoing internal work that extends far beyond therapy sessions. Once you learn to externalize internal conflicts and facilitate conversations between different parts of yourself, you have access to these skills whenever you need them. The chairs become internal resources that help you navigate life's challenges with greater wisdom and flexibility.

Essential Practice Elements

- Chair work externalizes internal conflicts through physical positioning and movement
- Basic two-chair setup provides the foundation for all chair work interventions
- Schema versus Healthy Adult dialogues strengthen adaptive responses to maladaptive patterns
- Empty chair work with absent figures helps resolve unfinished business and gain closure
- Inner critic confrontation builds immunity to self-attacking voices through direct challenge
- Parent-child chair work processes childhood relationships and their ongoing influence
- Mode-to-mode conversations improve internal communication and cooperation
- Relationship conflict practice builds skills and confidence for difficult real-world conversations
- Regular practice strengthens internal dialogue skills and emotional processing abilities

Chapter 6: Behavioral Pattern Breaking Exercises

Schemas don't just live in your thoughts and feelings—they express themselves through patterns of behavior that can persist for decades. You might intellectually understand that your perfectionism is unrealistic, but still find yourself staying late at work to revise projects that are already excellent. You might recognize your people-pleasing tendencies, yet continue saying yes to requests you don't want to fulfill. Behavioral pattern breaking bridges the gap between awareness and action, providing systematic approaches to changing the actions that keep schemas alive.

The challenge with behavioral change in schema work is that these patterns often serve important protective functions. Your avoidance behaviors might prevent anxiety in the short term, even as they limit your life in the long term. Your overcompensating behaviors might create temporary feelings of control, even as they exhaust you and damage relationships. Successful pattern breaking requires understanding what your behaviors accomplish before replacing them with healthier alternatives[21].

The exercises in this collection provide structured approaches to identifying problematic behavioral patterns, understanding their functions, and gradually replacing them with more adaptive responses. This work requires patience and self-compassion—these patterns developed over years and won't change overnight. But with consistent practice and appropriate support, even the most entrenched behavioral patterns can shift.

Exercise 34: Behavioral Pattern Breaking Worksheet

Planning Alternative Responses to Schema Triggers

The Behavioral Pattern Breaking Worksheet provides a systematic framework for identifying problematic behavioral responses to schema activation and developing healthier alternatives. This tool helps you move from automatic, schema-driven reactions to conscious, choice-based responses that serve your long-term wellbeing.

The worksheet works by breaking down behavioral patterns into their component parts: the trigger situation, the schema that gets activated, the typical behavioral response, the short-term consequences (what the behavior accomplishes), and the long-term costs (how the behavior creates problems). This analysis creates the foundation for developing alternative responses that meet the same needs more effectively.

Case Example: Janet's Conflict Avoidance Pattern

Janet, a 32-year-old nurse, used the worksheet to address her pattern of avoiding any form of interpersonal conflict. Her Abandonment schema created intense fear that disagreement would lead to rejection, causing her to suppress her own needs and opinions in both personal and professional relationships.

Janet's worksheet analysis revealed the following pattern:

Trigger Situation: Colleague suggests a patient care approach that Janet believes is suboptimal.

Schema Activated: Abandonment ("If I disagree, she'll think I'm difficult and won't want to work with me anymore")

Typical Behavioral Response: Say nothing, go along with the suggestion, handle any problems privately later.

Short-term Consequences: Avoids potential conflict, maintains appearance of agreeableness, reduces immediate anxiety.

Long-term Costs: Patient receives less optimal care, Janet feels frustrated and unheard, colleagues don't benefit from her expertise, her professional confidence erodes.

Alternative Response Options: Janet brainstormed several healthier alternatives:

1. Express disagreement diplomatically: "I have a different perspective on this approach. Could we discuss the options?"
2. Ask clarifying questions: "Help me understand your reasoning for this approach. I'm wondering about..."
3. Suggest collaboration: "What if we combined your idea with this modification?"

Implementation Plan: Janet chose to start with asking clarifying questions since this felt less threatening than direct disagreement. She practiced the phrases during calm moments and committed to using this approach in one low-stakes situation per week.

Results Tracking: After four weeks, Janet reported feeling more confident in professional discussions and receiving positive feedback from colleagues who appreciated her thoughtful questions. Her patient care improved as she became more engaged in treatment planning conversations.

Worksheet Implementation Guidelines

Start with specific behavioral patterns rather than general problems. "I avoid conflict" is too broad; "I don't speak up when colleagues suggest approaches I disagree with" is specific enough to work with.

Include both obvious behavioral responses (what others would observe) and subtle ones (internal reactions, body language, what you don't do).

Be honest about short-term benefits. Most problematic behaviors serve some protective function—acknowledging this reduces shame and resistance.

Brainstorm multiple alternative responses rather than trying to find the perfect solution. Having options reduces pressure and increases likelihood of follow-through.

Start with low-stakes situations for practicing new responses. Build confidence with easier scenarios before tackling more challenging ones.

Exercise 35: Coping Style Assessment

Identifying Surrender, Avoidance, and Overcompensation Patterns

Young identified three primary coping styles that people use in response to schema activation: surrender, avoidance, and overcompensation[22]. Understanding your dominant coping style provides essential information for targeting behavioral interventions effectively. Each style creates different types of problems and requires different approaches to change.

Surrender involves giving in to the schema and behaving as if it's completely true. Avoidance means organizing your life to prevent schema activation. Overcompensation involves acting in ways that directly oppose the schema, often to an extreme degree. Most people use all three styles at different times, but typically have one dominant pattern.

Case Example: Mark's Overcompensation Discovery

Mark, a 38-year-old sales manager, completed a coping style assessment and discovered that he primarily used overcompensation in response to his Defectiveness schema. Instead of surrendering to feelings of inadequacy or avoiding situations where he might be evaluated, Mark worked excessively hard to prove his worth and competence.

Mark's overcompensation patterns included:

- Working 12-hour days to ensure perfect performance
- Volunteering for every challenging project to demonstrate capability
- Constantly seeking praise and recognition from supervisors

- Becoming competitive and sometimes ruthless with colleagues
- Refusing to ask for help even when struggling
- Presenting a confident facade even when feeling overwhelmed

The assessment helped Mark understand that his "success-driven" behavior was actually a defensive response to deep feelings of inadequacy. His achievements felt hollow because they were motivated by schema avoidance rather than genuine interest or values.

Understanding his overcompensation pattern allowed Mark to recognize when he was pushing too hard and why. He began noticing the anxiety that drove his overwork and the emptiness that followed his achievements. This awareness created space for Mark to make different choices about how much effort was genuinely needed versus how much was schema-driven.

Mark developed specific strategies for moderating his overcompensation:

- Setting realistic work hours and sticking to them
- Choosing projects based on interest and growth rather than proving himself
- Practicing asking for help in low-stakes situations
- Celebrating achievements without immediately moving to the next challenge
- Taking time to rest without feeling guilty about "wasted" time

Assessment Implementation

Review multiple areas of life including work, relationships, social situations, and personal challenges. Coping styles often vary by context.

Look for patterns across time, not just current behavior. How did you handle similar schemas as a child, teenager, and young adult?

Include both behavioral responses and emotional/cognitive patterns. Surrender might involve self-critical thoughts, avoidance might include worrying, overcompensation might involve constant planning.

Consider the costs and benefits of each coping style in different situations. Sometimes avoidance is healthy, sometimes overcompensation is appropriate.

Identify which coping styles create the most problems in your current life circumstances. These become priorities for pattern breaking work.

Exercise 36: Assertiveness Training Scripts

Practicing New Communication Patterns

Assertiveness training provides specific language and approaches for expressing your needs, opinions, and boundaries in ways that are direct but respectful. For people with schemas like Subjugation, Self-Sacrifice, or Defectiveness, assertiveness often feels dangerous or impossible. These scripts provide concrete alternatives to passive, aggressive, or passive-aggressive communication patterns.

Effective assertiveness requires balancing honesty about your needs with respect for others' perspectives. The goal isn't getting your way all the time, but ensuring that your voice is heard and your needs are considered in decisions that affect you.

Case Example: Rachel's Boundary Setting Scripts

Rachel, a 30-year-old teacher, struggled with saying no to additional responsibilities at work. Her Self-Sacrifice schema made her feel obligated to help everyone, leading to overwhelming workloads and resentment toward colleagues who seemed to have better boundaries.

Rachel developed specific scripts for different boundary-setting situations:

For declining additional tasks: "I appreciate you thinking of me for this project. Unfortunately, I'm at capacity with my current responsibilities and can't take on anything additional right now."

For addressing unfair work distribution: "I've noticed that I've been assigned the last three weekend events while other teachers haven't had any. I'm wondering if we could distribute these more evenly going forward."

For responding to last-minute requests: "I understand this is urgent from your perspective. However, I have plans tonight that I can't change. I could help with this first thing tomorrow morning if that would work."

For offering alternatives when saying no: "I can't stay late to finish this today, but I could come in early tomorrow morning. Or perhaps Sarah would be available to help since she left early today."

Rachel practiced these scripts through role-playing with friends and rehearsing them mentally before potentially challenging conversations. She started with lower-stakes situations (declining to bring treats for a staff meeting) before moving to more significant boundaries (saying no to chaperoning weekend school events).

The scripts helped Rachel feel more confident because she had specific language to use instead of fumbling for words or giving in due to social pressure. Over time, she developed her own variations that felt natural while maintaining the assertive structure.

Script Development Process

Identify specific situations where you struggle with assertive communication. Create scripts for actual scenarios you face rather than hypothetical situations.

Include multiple options for each situation. People respond differently, so having several approaches increases your chances of successful communication.

Practice scripts out loud, not just mentally. Hearing yourself say the words helps build confidence and identifies awkward phrasing that needs revision.

Role-play with trusted friends or family members when possible. Practicing with real people helps you handle unexpected responses.

Start with written scripts but work toward more natural, conversational versions. The goal is internalized confidence, not memorized speeches.

Exercise 37: Boundary Setting Exercises

Learning to Say No and Protect Personal Limits

Boundary setting involves establishing and maintaining limits around your time, energy, emotions, and physical space. For people with schemas like Self-Sacrifice, Subjugation, or Approval-Seeking, boundaries often feel selfish or dangerous. These exercises provide graduated practice in setting healthy limits while maintaining important relationships.

Effective boundaries aren't walls that keep everyone out—they're doors with good locks that you control. The goal is protecting your wellbeing while remaining open to meaningful connection and appropriate requests for help.

Case Example: David's Energy Management Boundaries

David, a 35-year-old therapist, realized that his Emotional Deprivation schema was causing him to overextend himself professionally in hopes of receiving appreciation and connection. He would stay late to see additional clients, take calls from patients outside office hours, and volunteer for every committee that needed mental health representation.

David developed a systematic approach to boundary setting:

Time Boundaries:

- Set specific work hours and communicate them clearly to clients and colleagues

- Turn off work phone during personal time except for genuine emergencies
- Schedule breaks between clients and protect them from "quick questions"
- Limit work-related activities on weekends to two hours maximum

Emotional Boundaries:

- Stop taking personal responsibility for clients' progress between sessions
- Avoid giving friends and family members informal therapy outside relationships
- Set limits on how much work stress he discussed at home
- Practice saying "That sounds really difficult" instead of "What can I do to help?"

Physical Boundaries:

- Keep office door closed during documentation time
- Avoid hugging clients who initiated physical contact
- Take lunch breaks away from his office
- Set up his home office to be completely separate from living spaces

David implemented these boundaries gradually, starting with time limits that felt manageable. He discovered that clients respected his boundaries more than he expected, and colleagues didn't take his limits personally. His energy and enthusiasm for work actually increased as he felt more in control of his professional life.

Boundary Implementation Strategy

Start with boundaries that feel important but not terrifying. Build confidence with smaller limits before tackling major boundary challenges.

Communicate boundaries clearly and consistently. People can't respect limits they don't understand or that change unpredictably.

Expect some pushback, especially from people who have benefited from your previous lack of boundaries. This resistance doesn't mean your boundaries are wrong.

Prepare responses for boundary violations. "I understand you're disappointed, but I won't be able to change my decision about this."

Recognize that guilt about boundaries is normal, especially early in the process. Guilt doesn't mean you're doing something wrong—it often means you're changing a problematic pattern.

Exercise 38: Exposure Hierarchy for Schema Avoidance

Gradual Confrontation of Avoided Situations

Avoidance coping often involves organizing your entire life around preventing schema activation. While this can be effective in the short term, extensive avoidance typically limits your opportunities for growth, connection, and meaningful experience. Exposure hierarchy provides a systematic approach to gradually confronting avoided situations while building tolerance for schema-related discomfort.

The hierarchy works by listing avoided situations from least to most anxiety-provoking, then systematically working through them starting with the easiest. This gradual approach prevents overwhelming yourself while building confidence and tolerance.

Case Example: Lisa's Social Anxiety Hierarchy

Lisa, a 27-year-old graphic designer, had organized her life around avoiding situations that might trigger her Social Isolation and Defectiveness schemas. She worked from home, ordered groceries online, and declined most social invitations. While this avoided immediate anxiety, it reinforced her belief that she was fundamentally different from and inferior to others.

Lisa's exposure hierarchy included:

Level 1 (Least Anxiety-Provoking):

- Making eye contact with cashiers during necessary errands
- Saying "thank you" to service workers instead of just nodding
- Commenting on one social media post per week

Level 2:

- Asking questions in online work meetings
- Making small talk with neighbors when encountered
- Attending one public event per month (farmers market, library program)

Level 3:

- Initiating brief conversations with acquaintances
- Attending work-related social events for 30 minutes
- Joining one activity-based group (pottery class, hiking group)

Level 4:

- Expressing opinions that might differ from others'
- Inviting someone for coffee or lunch
- Attending parties and staying for more than an hour

Level 5 (Most Anxiety-Provoking):

- Hosting a small gathering at her home
- Going on dates and being authentic about her interests
- Speaking up in situations where she disagreed with group consensus

Lisa worked through her hierarchy over six months, spending 2-3 weeks on each level until her anxiety decreased significantly. She discovered that most people were more accepting and less judgmental than her schemas predicted. Her confidence grew with each successful exposure, creating positive momentum for tackling more challenging situations.

Hierarchy Development Guidelines

Include 8-12 items spanning the range from mildly uncomfortable to significantly anxiety-provoking. Too few items create large jumps in difficulty; too many can feel overwhelming.

Make items specific and behavioral rather than vague or emotional. "Have lunch with a coworker" is better than "be more social."

Ensure items are realistically achievable given your current life circumstances. The hierarchy should challenge you without being impossible.

Include both one-time activities and ongoing behavioral changes. Some exposures involve single actions while others require sustained practice.

Plan for setbacks and plateau periods. Progress isn't always linear, and some exposures may need to be repeated multiple times.

Exercise 39: Behavioral Experiments Planning

Testing New Behaviors Safely

Behavioral experiments involve testing new behaviors in controlled circumstances to gather evidence about their outcomes. This approach helps challenge schema-based predictions about what will happen if you change your patterns. Many schemas persist because they're never tested—you avoid the situations that might prove them wrong.

Effective experiments are designed like scientific studies with clear hypotheses, specific measurements, and objective evaluation of results. This structure helps separate schema-based fears from actual evidence about what happens when you try new behaviors.

Case Example: Tom's Perfectionism Experiments

Tom, a 41-year-old accountant, wanted to test his Unrelenting Standards schema's prediction that anything less than perfect work would result in criticism and professional failure. His schema insisted that he needed to check his work multiple times and stay late to ensure absolute accuracy.

Tom designed several behavioral experiments:

Experiment 1: Submit a report after checking it twice instead of his usual five times.

- **Hypothesis**: The report will contain errors that damage my reputation
- **Prediction**: My supervisor will criticize the work and question my competence
- **Measurement**: Track any errors found and supervisor feedback
- **Actual Result**: No errors were found, supervisor praised the timely submission

Experiment 2: Leave work at normal hours instead of staying late to perfect tomorrow's presentation.

- **Hypothesis**: The presentation will be inadequate and embarrassing
- **Prediction**: Colleagues will notice the lower quality and think less of me
- **Measurement**: Presentation feedback and audience engagement
- **Actual Result**: Presentation went well, several colleagues asked follow-up questions

Experiment 3: Ask for clarification on a project instead of spending hours trying to figure it out alone.

- **Hypothesis**: Asking questions reveals incompetence and burdens colleagues
- **Prediction**: Supervisor will be annoyed and doubt my abilities

- **Measurement**: Supervisor's response and subsequent interactions
- **Actual Result**: Supervisor appreciated the initiative and provided helpful guidance

These experiments helped Tom recognize that his perfectionist behaviors were unnecessary and often counterproductive. His work quality remained high while his stress decreased significantly. The evidence contradicted his schema's predictions and supported more balanced work habits.

Experiment Design Process

Choose behaviors that directly test your schema's predictions rather than unrelated activities. The goal is gathering relevant evidence about your specific fears.

Start with lower-risk experiments that won't create serious problems if your schema's predictions are accurate. Build confidence before tackling higher-stakes tests.

Define success clearly before conducting the experiment. What outcome would prove your schema wrong? What would confirm its predictions?

Include multiple measurements when possible. Look at both objective outcomes (what actually happened) and subjective responses (how you felt, what you learned).

Plan follow-up experiments that build on initial results. One successful test doesn't eliminate a schema, but multiple successes create compelling evidence for change.

Exercise 40: Relapse Prevention for Old Patterns

Maintaining New Behavioral Changes

Behavioral change rarely follows a straight line from old patterns to new ones. Setbacks, stress periods, and challenging life circumstances can trigger returns to familiar schema-driven behaviors. Relapse prevention involves anticipating these challenges and developing strategies for maintaining progress during difficult times.

The goal isn't preventing all setbacks—that's unrealistic and creates additional pressure. Instead, relapse prevention focuses on recognizing setbacks early, responding to them skillfully, and getting back on track quickly without shame or abandonment of new patterns.

Case Example: Sarah's People-Pleasing Recovery Plan

Sarah, a 29-year-old marketing coordinator, had made significant progress in reducing her Self-Sacrifice schema behaviors. She was saying no to unreasonable requests, setting boundaries with demanding clients, and prioritizing her own needs more consistently. However, she recognized that certain situations triggered returns to her old people-pleasing patterns.

Sarah's relapse prevention plan included:

High-Risk Situations:

- Family gatherings where relatives made excessive demands
- Work deadline periods when everyone felt stressed
- Relationship conflicts where she feared abandonment
- Times when she felt lonely or disconnected from others

Early Warning Signs:

- Saying yes immediately without considering her capacity
- Feeling resentful but not expressing her needs
- Working through lunch breaks and evenings without compensation
- Avoiding people rather than setting appropriate boundaries

Emergency Strategies:

- 24-hour rule: "Let me check my schedule and get back to you tomorrow"
- Support person check-ins: calling her sister when feeling pressured to overcommit
- Values reminder: reviewing her priorities when feeling pulled to people-please
- Self-compassion practice: treating setbacks as learning opportunities, not failures

Recovery Strategies:

- Honest communication: explaining to others when she'd overcommitted and needed to adjust
- Boundary reset: implementing limits that should have been in place initially
- Energy restoration: taking time to recover from periods of over-giving
- Pattern analysis: understanding what triggered the relapse to prevent future occurrences

Sarah's plan helped her navigate several challenging periods without completely abandoning her new boundaries. When she did slip back into people-pleasing patterns, she recovered more quickly and learned from each experience.

Prevention Planning Elements

Identify your specific high-risk situations based on past experience. When are you most likely to return to old patterns?

Develop early warning systems that help you recognize the beginning of relapse rather than waiting until patterns are fully reestablished.

Create multiple intervention strategies for different levels of risk. Small slips need different responses than major setbacks.

Include self-compassion practices in your prevention plan. Shame about setbacks often leads to abandoning change efforts entirely.

Build support systems that can help you maintain perspective during challenging periods. Include both professional and personal sources of encouragement.

Moving From Awareness to Action

Behavioral pattern breaking represents the bridge between understanding your schemas and creating lasting change in your daily life. All the awareness and emotional processing in the world won't change your experience if your behaviors continue reinforcing old patterns. These exercises provide systematic approaches to translating insight into action.

The work requires patience, self-compassion, and realistic expectations. Behavioral patterns that have persisted for years or decades won't change overnight. However, even small shifts in behavior can create significant changes in how you feel about yourself and how others respond to you.

Success in behavioral change often creates positive feedback loops that support continued growth. As you experience the benefits of healthier patterns—better relationships, reduced anxiety, increased self-respect—motivation for maintaining new behaviors increases naturally. The behaviors that once felt foreign and difficult become more automatic and comfortable over time.

Practice Principles for Success

- Behavioral pattern breaking requires systematic planning and gradual implementation
- Understanding the protective functions of old patterns reduces resistance to change
- Coping style assessment reveals whether you tend toward surrender, avoidance, or overcompensation patterns
- Assertiveness training provides concrete language for expressing needs and maintaining boundaries
- Boundary setting protects your time, energy, and emotional wellbeing while preserving relationships

- Exposure hierarchy allows gradual confrontation of avoided situations without overwhelming yourself
- Behavioral experiments test schema predictions against actual evidence through controlled trials
- Relapse prevention planning helps maintain progress during challenging periods and stressful life circumstances
- Sustainable change balances pushing for growth with accepting temporary setbacks as part of the process

Chapter 7: Cognitive Restructuring and Thought Records

Your thoughts shape your reality more than you might realize. The running commentary in your mind—about yourself, others, and the world around you—creates the emotional tone of your experience and influences every decision you make. Schema-driven thoughts operate like background software, automatically interpreting events through the lens of your earliest learning about relationships, safety, and self-worth. Cognitive restructuring provides tools for updating this mental software when it no longer serves your wellbeing.

Unlike traditional cognitive therapy that focuses primarily on surface-level thoughts, schema-focused cognitive work addresses the deeper belief systems that generate automatic thoughts. A person might successfully challenge the thought "I'm going to fail this presentation" while never addressing the underlying Failure schema that creates such thoughts repeatedly. The exercises in this section target both levels—the immediate thoughts that create distress and the fundamental beliefs that create those thoughts[23].

The goal isn't to eliminate all negative thinking or create unrealistic positivity. Instead, cognitive restructuring helps you develop more balanced, accurate, and helpful ways of thinking about yourself and your experiences. This work requires patience and practice—schemas have been shaping your thoughts for years, and they won't change their patterns overnight.

Exercise 41: Schema-Focused Thought Record

Identifying and Challenging Schema-Driven Thoughts

The Schema-Focused Thought Record expands traditional thought records by explicitly connecting automatic thoughts to their underlying schema patterns. This tool helps you recognize when your thinking is being influenced by old wounds rather than current realities, creating space for more balanced and accurate interpretations of events.

Standard thought records often address thoughts in isolation, missing the deeper patterns that connect seemingly unrelated negative thoughts. Schema-focused records reveal these patterns, making it easier to address the root causes rather than just the symptoms of distorted thinking.

Case Example: Amanda's Perfectionist Thought Patterns

Amanda, a 33-year-old lawyer, used schema-focused thought records to address the constant stream of self-critical thoughts that accompanied her daily work. Her Unrelenting Standards schema generated multiple negative thoughts throughout each day, creating chronic stress and undermining her confidence despite her professional success.

Situation: Received feedback from senior partner suggesting minor revisions to a brief

Automatic Thoughts:

- "I should have caught those issues myself"
- "A good lawyer wouldn't need this kind of basic feedback"
- "She probably thinks I'm incompetent"
- "I'm not ready for this level of responsibility"

Emotions: Shame (8/10), Anxiety (7/10), Discouragement (6/10)

Schema Identified: Unrelenting Standards ("I must be perfect or I'm worthless")

Schema-Driven Thinking Patterns:

- All-or-nothing thinking: One piece of feedback means complete incompetence
- Mind reading: Assuming supervisor's thoughts without evidence

- Impossible standards: Expecting perfection on first drafts
- Personalization: Taking responsibility for normal learning process

Balanced Response: "This feedback is actually helpful and shows my supervisor is invested in my development. All lawyers receive feedback on their work—that's how the profession maintains quality. The suggested revisions are minor and will make the brief stronger. I'm learning and improving, which is exactly what I should be doing at this stage of my career."

Evidence For Balanced Thoughts:

- Senior partner specifically requested me for this case
- Previous work has received positive feedback
- Colleagues regularly discuss receiving and incorporating feedback
- The brief's main arguments were solid; only minor improvements suggested

Schema Challenge: "The Unrelenting Standards schema tells me that needing feedback means I'm failing, but the evidence shows that feedback is a normal part of professional development. I can strive for excellence without demanding perfection from myself."

Amanda's thought records revealed consistent patterns where her schema created catastrophic interpretations of normal professional interactions. Tracking these patterns helped her recognize schema activation earlier and develop more realistic responses.

Implementation Guidelines

Complete thought records as soon after emotional reactions as possible. Fresh memories provide more accurate information about thoughts and feelings.

Include both the automatic thoughts that popped into your mind and the deeper beliefs they reflect. Look for the schema themes underlying multiple thoughts.

Rate emotional intensity before and after challenging thoughts. This helps track the effectiveness of cognitive work over time.

Focus on accuracy rather than positivity. The goal is realistic thinking, not optimistic thinking that ignores legitimate concerns.

Look for patterns across multiple thought records. Are the same schemas generating thoughts repeatedly? What situations most commonly trigger schema-driven thinking?

Exercise 42: Evidence For/Against Schema Beliefs

Rational Evaluation of Core Beliefs

Evidence gathering provides a systematic approach to evaluating the accuracy of schema-driven beliefs. This exercise helps you step back from the emotional intensity of schema activation and examine your core beliefs with the same objectivity you might use to evaluate evidence in other contexts.

Schemas often persist because they're never subjected to careful evaluation. They feel true because they've been with you for so long, not because they accurately reflect your current reality. Evidence gathering creates opportunities to test these beliefs against actual life experience.

Case Example: Martin's Defectiveness Belief Examination

Martin, a 39-year-old teacher, struggled with a deep belief that something was fundamentally wrong with him that others would discover if they got to know him well. His Defectiveness schema created chronic anxiety in relationships and prevented him from forming close friendships or romantic partnerships.

Core Schema Belief: "I am fundamentally flawed and unworthy of love. If people really knew me, they would reject me."

Evidence That Seems to Support This Belief:

- Relationship ended in college when girlfriend said we "weren't compatible"
- Sometimes feel awkward in social situations
- Parents were often critical during childhood
- Don't have as many close friends as some people seem to have
- Worry about saying the wrong thing in conversations

Evidence Against This Belief:

- Students consistently rate me as their favorite teacher
- Colleagues regularly seek my advice and collaboration
- Sister calls me frequently and values my support
- Friends from childhood still stay in contact after 20+ years
- Neighbors trust me to care for their pets and homes when they travel
- Multiple students have written thank-you notes mentioning my positive impact
- Book club members seem to enjoy my participation and insights
- Running club teammates invited me to social events outside running
- Former students sometimes contact me years later to share their successes

Alternative, More Balanced Belief: "Like everyone, I have both strengths and areas for growth. Some people will connect with me while others won't, and that's normal in all relationships. The evidence shows that many people value my friendship, mentorship, and collaboration. I am worthy of love and connection, even though I sometimes feel insecure about my relationships."

Behavioral Test of New Belief: Martin committed to having lunch with a colleague he'd been wanting to know better, joining one social event per month, and sharing more personal information in existing friendships to test whether people would accept or reject the "real" him.

The evidence gathering helped Martin recognize how selectively his schema had been filtering information, focusing on limited negative experiences while ignoring extensive positive evidence about his worth and lovability.

Evidence Evaluation Process

Write down the schema belief in specific, clear language. Vague beliefs are harder to evaluate than precise statements.

Gather evidence systematically rather than relying on memory alone. Review journals, photos, emails, or other records that might provide objective information.

Include both current evidence and historical patterns. Sometimes schemas are based on past experiences that are no longer relevant to current circumstances.

Ask trusted friends or family members for their perspectives. Others can often see strengths and positive qualities that schemas make invisible to you.

Consider behavioral experiments that could provide additional evidence. What actions would test the accuracy of your schema beliefs?

Exercise 43: Schema Dialogue Worksheet

Written Conversations Between Different Perspectives

Schema dialogue worksheets create structured written conversations between your schema voice and your healthy adult voice, allowing both perspectives to express themselves fully before working toward balanced conclusions. Writing these dialogues helps you externalize internal conflicts and develop stronger healthy responses to schema activation.

Unlike spoken dialogues that happen in real time, written conversations allow for more careful consideration of each perspective and the development of thoughtful responses. The written format also creates a record that can be reviewed later for patterns and progress.

Case Example: Rebecca's Self-Sacrifice Dialogue

Rebecca, a 35-year-old social worker, used dialogue worksheets to address internal conflicts between her Self-Sacrifice schema and her need for personal boundaries and self-care.

Schema Voice: "You can't say no to covering Sarah's shift this weekend. She's having family problems, and she's always been nice to you. If you don't help, she'll think you're selfish, and other people will see that you only care about yourself. Good people sacrifice for others, especially when they're going through difficult times."

Healthy Adult Voice: "I understand you want me to be a caring person who helps others, and that's an important value for me too. But I've already covered three extra shifts this month, and I have my own commitments this weekend. Saying no to one request doesn't make me selfish—it makes me human with reasonable limits."

Schema Voice: "But you don't have anything really important planned. You're just going to relax and spend time with friends. That's not as important as helping someone in need. You should be grateful you have a job and willing to do whatever it takes to support your coworkers."

Healthy Adult Voice: "Rest and friendship are important for my wellbeing, not frivolous luxuries. I'm a better social worker and colleague when I'm not exhausted and resentful. There are other ways to support Sarah—I could help her find another person to cover the shift, or offer to listen if she needs to talk about her family situation."

Schema Voice: "You're just making excuses because you're lazy and don't want to make the effort. Really caring people don't think about themselves first."

Healthy Adult Voice: "Taking care of my own needs isn't laziness—it's responsibility. I can't take care of others effectively if I'm burned out and resentful. Setting this boundary allows me to continue being helpful when it's genuinely needed and when I have the energy to give freely."

Resolution: "I will offer to help Sarah find someone else to cover the shift and let her know I'm available to talk if she needs emotional support. I will maintain my weekend plans and use the time to recharge so I can be more present and helpful in the future."

The dialogue process helped Rebecca recognize how her schema created guilt about normal self-care while developing stronger rationales for maintaining healthy boundaries.

Dialogue Development Process

Let each voice express itself fully before responding. Avoid cutting off the schema voice too quickly or dismissing its concerns without consideration.

Use the natural language each voice employs. Schema voices often use words like "should," "always," "never," while healthy voices tend to be more flexible and nuanced.

Include both emotional and logical arguments. Schemas aren't purely irrational, and healthy responses need to address both feeling and thinking.

Work toward resolution that honors both perspectives when possible. Sometimes the schema voice has legitimate concerns that need addressing in healthier ways.

Practice dialogues regularly, not just during crisis moments. Developing the healthy voice requires consistent exercise and strengthening.

Exercise 44: Cognitive Distortions in Schemas

Identifying Thinking Errors

Schemas often operate through specific cognitive distortions—systematic errors in thinking that create negative interpretations of neutral or positive events. Identifying these distortions helps you recognize when your thinking is being influenced by schema patterns rather than accurate perception of reality.

Common distortions in schema-driven thinking include all-or-nothing thinking, mind reading, fortune telling, emotional reasoning, and personalization. Learning to spot these patterns creates opportunities to question and revise automatic interpretations of events.

Case Example: Kevin's Social Anxiety Distortions

Kevin, a 28-year-old graphic designer, identified multiple cognitive distortions that maintained his Social Isolation and Defectiveness schemas. His thinking patterns consistently interpreted social interactions negatively, reinforcing his belief that he was different from and inferior to others.

All-or-Nothing Thinking:

- Distortion: "If I say something awkward at this party, the entire evening will be ruined"
- Challenge: "Conversations naturally include some awkward moments. One comment doesn't determine the whole interaction"

Mind Reading:

- Distortion: "She's looking at her phone, so she must be bored by our conversation"
- Challenge: "There are many reasons people check phones. I don't actually know what she's thinking"

Fortune Telling:

- Distortion: "If I go to this networking event, I'll embarrass myself and damage my professional reputation"
- Challenge: "I don't know what will happen. I've had successful professional conversations before"

Emotional Reasoning:

- Distortion: "I feel anxious about calling him, so he probably doesn't want to hear from me"
- Challenge: "My anxiety comes from my schema, not from evidence about his feelings"

Personalization:

- Distortion: "The group got quiet when I joined the conversation, so they must not want me there"
- Challenge: "Group dynamics change for many reasons. Their reaction might have nothing to do with me"

Mental Filter:

- Distortion: Focusing only on the one person who didn't respond to his greeting while ignoring five people who smiled and said hello
- Challenge: "I'm filtering out positive responses and focusing only on neutral ones"

Learning to identify these distortions helped Kevin catch schema-driven thinking in real time and develop more balanced interpretations of social interactions. His social anxiety decreased as his thinking became more accurate and realistic.

Distortion Identification Process

Learn the common cognitive distortions and their definitions. Understanding the categories helps you recognize patterns in your own thinking.

Track distortions in a journal or thought record for several weeks. Look for patterns in which distortions you use most frequently.

Practice identifying distortions in low-stakes situations before working on emotionally charged events. Build the skill when you're calm and thinking clearly.

Question the evidence for thoughts that seem to involve distortions. What proof do you have for this interpretation? What other explanations are possible?

Develop standard challenges for your most common distortions. Having prepared responses makes it easier to challenge distorted thinking in the moment.

Exercise 45: Healthy Adult Response Generator

Developing Adaptive Self-Talk

The Healthy Adult Response Generator helps you develop specific language and perspectives that counteract schema-driven thoughts and emotions. This exercise focuses on building an internal voice that is wise, balanced, compassionate, and realistic—qualities that can guide you through difficult situations without being overwhelmed by schema patterns.

Effective healthy adult responses acknowledge legitimate concerns while providing perspective and practical guidance. They neither dismiss emotions nor get lost in them, creating a middle path between schema extremes and unrealistic positivity.

Case Example: Jennifer's Abandonment Response Development

Jennifer, a 31-year-old nurse, developed healthy adult responses to counteract her Abandonment schema's catastrophic interpretations of relationship events. Her schema created intense anxiety whenever her boyfriend seemed distant or unavailable, flooding her with fears of imminent rejection.

Schema Trigger: Boyfriend seems quieter than usual during dinner

Schema Response: "He's losing interest in me. This is how it starts—first they become distant, then they find excuses to spend less time together, then they leave. I need to figure out what I did wrong and fix it before he decides to break up with me."

Healthy Adult Response: "Tom seems preoccupied tonight, and there could be many reasons for that. He mentioned having a difficult day at work, so he might just be processing stress. Our relationship has been stable and loving for eight months—one quiet evening doesn't indicate a fundamental change. I can ask if he wants to talk about his day, or simply give him space to work through whatever he's dealing with."

Schema Trigger: Boyfriend doesn't respond to text for several hours

Schema Response: "He's avoiding me. This is probably his way of pulling back without having to have an awkward conversation. I should text again to see if he got my message, or maybe call to make sure everything is okay."

Healthy Adult Response: "Four hours isn't an unusual time to wait for a text response, especially during work hours. Tom has consistently responded to my messages throughout our relationship—there's no pattern of avoidance or pulling away. I can wait for his response without needing to follow up immediately. If I don't hear from him by tomorrow, I can check in casually."

Schema Trigger: Plans to see each other get cancelled due to his work obligation

Schema Response: "He's making excuses to avoid spending time with me. Work is becoming more important than our relationship. This is how people start creating distance before they end things."

Healthy Adult Response: "Work obligations sometimes interfere with personal plans—that's normal in adult relationships. Tom seemed genuinely disappointed about cancelling, and he immediately suggested alternative times we could get together. His job requires occasional weekend work, and he's been transparent about this from the beginning of our relationship."

These healthy responses helped Jennifer respond to relationship anxiety with perspective rather than panic, strengthening her relationship rather than creating the problems her schema feared.

Response Development Guidelines

Create responses that are specific to your most common schema triggers rather than generic positive affirmations. Personalized responses feel more authentic and convincing.

Include both emotional validation and rational perspective. Acknowledge that your schema's concerns make sense given your history while providing current evidence.

Use language that feels natural and believable to you. Responses that sound foreign or forced won't be effective when you're emotionally activated.

Practice responses during calm moments so they're available during stress. Reading healthy responses when you're already overwhelmed is less effective than having them readily accessible.

Update responses as you gather new evidence and experiences. Healthy responses should evolve as your understanding and confidence grow.

Exercise 46: Schema Cost-Benefit Analysis

Evaluating Pros and Cons of Schema Patterns

Schema cost-benefit analysis provides a systematic evaluation of what your schemas accomplish versus what they cost you. This exercise helps you understand why schemas persist—they often provide real benefits, at least in the short term. Understanding these benefits is essential for developing alternative strategies that meet the same needs more effectively.

Schemas rarely persist solely because of habit or ignorance. They continue operating because they serve important functions: protection from pain, maintenance of familiar identity, or achievement of certain goals. Acknowledging these benefits reduces resistance to change while highlighting the need for alternative approaches.

Case Example: Michael's Perfectionism Analysis

Michael, a 37-year-old marketing director, conducted a cost-benefit analysis of his Unrelenting Standards schema to understand why it felt so difficult to moderate his perfectionist tendencies despite recognizing their costs.

Benefits of Unrelenting Standards Schema:

- Produces high-quality work that receives recognition and praise
- Prevents most mistakes and their associated embarrassment or criticism
- Creates sense of control in uncertain situations
- Maintains professional reputation and competitive advantage
- Provides clear standards for evaluating progress and success
- Motivates consistent effort and prevents complacency
- Aligns with family values about hard work and achievement

Costs of Unrelenting Standards Schema:

- Creates chronic stress and anxiety about performance
- Leads to working excessive hours and missing family time
- Generates harsh self-criticism when standards aren't met

- Prevents delegation and team development
- Creates unrealistic expectations for colleagues and family members
- Interferes with creativity by making risk-taking feel dangerous
- Causes procrastination when tasks feel too important to do imperfectly
- Undermines satisfaction with achievements by immediately raising standards

Alternative Strategies That Preserve Benefits While Reducing Costs:

- Set "good enough" standards for routine tasks while maintaining high standards for truly important projects
- Build review processes that catch errors without requiring personal perfection
- Develop team members' skills so delegation becomes possible without quality concerns
- Create specific time boundaries that force prioritization and prevent endless revision
- Practice self-compassion when mistakes occur while still learning from them
- Schedule regular breaks and personal time as non-negotiable appointments

The analysis helped Michael recognize that his perfectionism wasn't purely destructive—it had genuinely contributed to his professional success. This understanding reduced his resistance to change while highlighting the need for more sustainable approaches to maintaining quality.

Analysis Implementation Process

Be honest about the real benefits your schemas provide, even if they seem negative or unhealthy. Denying benefits makes change more difficult.

Include both obvious costs and subtle ones. Schemas often create hidden costs in relationships, creativity, or life satisfaction that are easy to overlook.

Consider short-term versus long-term consequences. Some schema benefits are immediate while their costs accumulate over time.

Involve trusted others in identifying costs you might not recognize. Schemas can create blind spots about their impact on relationships and opportunities.

Use the analysis to guide alternative strategy development rather than simply trying to eliminate schema patterns entirely.

Exercise 47: Reframing Exercises

Creating Alternative Interpretations of Events

Reframing involves developing alternative interpretations of events that activate your schemas, creating more balanced and helpful perspectives on difficult situations. This technique recognizes that events themselves are often neutral—their emotional impact comes from how we interpret and understand them.

Effective reframing doesn't involve denying problems or creating false optimism. Instead, it expands your perspective to include possibilities that your schemas might filter out, leading to more flexible and adaptive responses to challenging situations.

Case Example: Carol's Rejection Reframing

Carol, a 32-year-old writer, worked on reframing experiences of rejection that activated her Defectiveness and Failure schemas. Professional rejections from publishers and literary magazines consistently triggered intense shame and thoughts about giving up writing entirely.

Original Interpretation: "The magazine rejected my story because it's not good enough. I'm not a real writer, and I'm fooling myself by continuing to submit my work. This rejection proves that I don't have talent and should find a different career path."

Reframed Interpretations:

Perspective 1 - Market Fit: "This magazine might not be the right fit for my style or genre. They receive hundreds of submissions and can only publish a few pieces each month. Rejection often reflects editorial needs and preferences rather than quality judgments."

Perspective 2 - Growth Opportunity: "Rejection is part of every writer's journey and provides information about how to improve. Even published authors collect rejection letters—it's evidence that I'm putting my work out there rather than keeping it hidden."

Perspective 3 - Timing and Context: "The timing might not be right for this particular piece. Magazines have themes, seasonal considerations, and space limitations that affect selection. My story might be excellent but not what they need right now."

Perspective 4 - Volume and Persistence: "Professional writers submit their work widely and expect most submissions to be rejected. Success comes from persistent effort and multiple submissions, not from avoiding rejection entirely."

Balanced Integration: "While this rejection is disappointing, it doesn't provide evidence about my overall ability as a writer. I can use any feedback provided to improve the story, research other publications that might be better fits, and continue developing my skills through writing and submission practice."

The reframing exercises helped Carol maintain motivation and perspective during the inevitable rejections that come with pursuing creative work, preventing schema activation from derailing her writing goals.

Reframing Development Process

Start with specific triggering events rather than trying to reframe general life circumstances. Concrete situations are easier to work with than abstract concerns.

Generate multiple alternative interpretations rather than searching for the "right" one. Having options provides flexibility for different situations.

Include perspectives that other people might have about the same event. Friends, family members, or colleagues might see aspects you miss.

Consider both situational factors (timing, context, other people's circumstances) and personal growth opportunities in your reframes.

Test reframes against available evidence. Effective reframes should be plausible and supportive while remaining grounded in reality.

Thinking Your Way to Freedom

Cognitive restructuring provides essential tools for changing the mental patterns that maintain schema activation and emotional distress. By learning to recognize, evaluate, and modify schema-driven thoughts, you can create more balanced and helpful internal dialogues that support your wellbeing and growth.

The work requires consistent practice and patience—thought patterns that have operated for years don't change overnight. However, every time you catch a schema-driven thought and respond with a more balanced perspective, you're creating new neural pathways that support healthier thinking patterns. Over time, these healthier responses become more automatic and accessible.

The goal isn't to eliminate all negative thoughts or create unrealistic optimism. Instead, cognitive restructuring helps you develop mental flexibility—the ability to consider multiple perspectives, evaluate evidence objectively, and choose thoughts that serve your wellbeing rather than reinforcing old wounds.

Success in cognitive work often creates positive cycles that support continued growth. As your thinking becomes more balanced and realistic, your emotional reactions become less intense and your behavioral choices become more conscious. This creates opportunities for experiences that contradict schema predictions, providing additional evidence for healthier beliefs about yourself and your relationships.

Reflection on Understanding

Cognitive restructuring represents the meeting point between awareness and action in schema healing work. You can understand your schemas emotionally and process them experientially, but lasting change requires updating the moment-to-moment thoughts that maintain these patterns in daily life.

The exercises in this section provide systematic approaches to recognizing and changing the thinking patterns that keep schemas alive. Whether through thought records, evidence gathering, or reframing techniques, each tool helps you step back from automatic reactions and choose more conscious responses to life's challenges.

The most powerful aspect of cognitive work may be its immediacy— these tools are available whenever schema-driven thoughts arise. You don't need a therapy session or perfect circumstances to practice challenging distorted thinking or generating healthier responses. Your mind becomes the laboratory for transformation, with each difficult moment providing opportunities to practice new ways of thinking about yourself and your experiences.

Essential Elements for Transformation

- Schema-focused thought records connect automatic thoughts to underlying belief patterns for deeper understanding
- Evidence gathering tests schema beliefs against actual life experience rather than emotional conviction
- Written dialogues externalize internal conflicts and strengthen healthy adult responses through practice

- Cognitive distortion identification reveals systematic thinking errors that maintain schema patterns
- Healthy adult response development builds internal wisdom and perspective for handling difficult situations
- Cost-benefit analysis acknowledges schema functions while highlighting needs for alternative strategies
- Reframing exercises expand interpretive flexibility and reduce emotional reactivity to triggering events
- Consistent practice creates new mental habits that gradually replace schema-driven thinking patterns
- Cognitive flexibility allows conscious choice about which thoughts to follow and which to question

Chapter 8: Emotion Regulation and Self-Soothing Tools

Emotions can feel like wild horses—powerful, unpredictable, and sometimes overwhelming in their intensity. Schema activation often floods your nervous system with feelings that seem too big for your current situation, as if your eight-year-old self is reacting to today's challenges with yesterday's terror or rage. Learning to regulate these emotional storms while honoring their messages represents one of the most essential skills in schema healing work.

Traditional therapy often focuses on understanding emotions or changing thoughts about them, but schema work requires more direct engagement with your emotional and nervous system responses. Your body carries the imprints of early experiences, and healing requires tools that address these somatic patterns alongside cognitive and behavioral changes. The exercises in this section provide practical approaches to managing emotional intensity while building your capacity for emotional resilience and flexibility[40].

Emotion regulation doesn't mean suppressing or eliminating difficult feelings. Instead, it involves developing the skills to experience emotions fully without being overwhelmed by them, to express them appropriately without damaging relationships, and to use their information wisely without being controlled by their urgency. These tools help you become the skilled rider of those emotional horses rather than their helpless passenger.

Exercise 48: Emotional Needs Assessment

Identifying and Addressing Core Emotional Needs

Human beings enter the world with universal emotional needs that remain constant throughout life: safety, connection, autonomy, competence, meaning, and authenticity[41]. When these needs go unmet—either in childhood or currently—they create emotional disturbance that often manifests as schema activation. The Emotional

Needs Assessment helps identify which needs require attention and develops strategies for meeting them in healthy, age-appropriate ways.

Unlike physical needs that signal their absence clearly (hunger, thirst, fatigue), emotional needs often express themselves indirectly through mood changes, relationship difficulties, or compulsive behaviors. Learning to recognize and address these needs directly reduces the likelihood of schema activation while improving overall life satisfaction.

Case Example: Sarah's Connection Hunger

Sarah, a 31-year-old marketing manager, experienced frequent episodes of anxiety and depression that seemed unrelated to external circumstances. Her life looked successful from the outside—good job, nice apartment, financial stability—but she felt empty and restless most of the time. The Emotional Needs Assessment revealed that her need for authentic connection was severely unmet.

Sarah's assessment showed adequate meeting of safety needs (financial security, stable housing), competence needs (professional success, skill development), and autonomy needs (independent living, career choices). However, her scores for connection needs were extremely low. She had many acquaintances but no close friendships, dated occasionally but avoided emotional intimacy, and maintained only superficial contact with family members.

The assessment revealed that Sarah's Emotional Deprivation and Mistrust schemas were creating a double bind: she desperately needed connection but feared the vulnerability required to create it. Her strategies for protecting herself from potential hurt were preventing her from getting the emotional nourishment she craved.

Sarah developed specific action plans for meeting her connection needs:

- Joining a book club to practice regular social interaction around shared interests

- Scheduling monthly phone calls with her sister to rebuild family relationships
- Practicing vulnerability in small doses by sharing more personal information with trusted colleagues
- Considering therapy as a safe space to practice emotional connection
- Setting a goal of developing one close friendship within the next year

As Sarah began meeting her connection needs more directly, her general anxiety decreased and her mood stabilized. She discovered that much of her emotional distress stemmed from unmet needs rather than inherent psychological problems.

Assessment Implementation Process

Rate your current satisfaction with each core emotional need on a scale of 1-10, considering both frequency (how often the need gets met) and quality (how well it gets met when it does occur).

For safety needs, consider both physical safety (security, protection from harm) and emotional safety (predictability, trust, freedom from chronic stress). For connection needs, evaluate both quantity (how many meaningful relationships you have) and depth (how emotionally intimate and supportive they are).

Autonomy needs include both external freedom (making your own choices, controlling your environment) and internal autonomy (knowing your preferences, trusting your judgment, expressing your authentic self). Competence needs involve feeling effective and skilled in areas that matter to you.

Meaning needs relate to feeling that your life has purpose, that your actions matter, and that you're contributing to something larger than yourself. Authenticity needs involve being able to express your true thoughts, feelings, and personality without excessive fear of judgment or rejection.

Identify the 2-3 needs with the lowest scores and develop specific, actionable plans for addressing them. Focus on small, consistent actions rather than dramatic life changes that might be unsustainable.

Exercise 49: Self-Soothing Techniques Menu

Personalized Comfort Strategies

Self-soothing involves activating your nervous system's natural calming responses through intentional engagement with comforting sensory experiences, thoughts, or activities. These techniques help you manage emotional intensity in the moment while building your overall capacity for emotional regulation. The key is developing a personalized menu of strategies that work reliably for your specific nervous system and life circumstances.

Effective self-soothing engages multiple senses and addresses different types of distress. Some techniques work better for anxiety, others for sadness or anger. Some are appropriate for public settings, others require privacy. Building a diverse repertoire ensures you have options regardless of the situation or type of emotional activation you're experiencing.

Case Example: Marcus's Trauma Recovery Toolkit

Marcus, a 34-year-old paramedic, struggled with emotional flashbacks and hypervigilance related to both childhood trauma and work-related stress. His nervous system often felt stuck in high alert, making it difficult to relax even during time off. The self-soothing menu helped him develop specific techniques for different types of emotional activation.

For anxiety and hypervigilance, Marcus developed visual soothing techniques: looking at photos of peaceful nature scenes on his phone, watching fish in his aquarium, and practicing soft gaze meditation where he relaxed his eyes and peripheral vision. These activities helped activate his parasympathetic nervous system and reduce the intensity of his surveillance behaviors.

For anger and frustration, Marcus used physical soothing: taking hot showers, doing progressive muscle relaxation, and squeezing and releasing a stress ball while breathing deeply. These techniques helped him discharge physical tension without expressing anger inappropriately at work or home.

For sadness and grief, Marcus employed nurturing activities: listening to specific playlists that matched and then gradually shifted his mood, wrapping himself in a weighted blanket, and calling his sister for emotional support. These activities provided comfort without trying to eliminate the feelings entirely.

For general stress relief, Marcus used scent-based soothing: keeping lavender essential oil in his car, burning specific candles during his evening routine, and using eucalyptus shower melts to create a spa-like experience at home. These scents became anchors that signaled safety and relaxation to his nervous system.

Marcus practiced these techniques during calm moments to strengthen the neural pathways before trying to use them during emotional crises. Over time, he could access calming responses more quickly and effectively during stressful situations.

Menu Development Guidelines

Include techniques for all five senses: visual (calming images, nature scenes, soft lighting), auditory (music, nature sounds, guided meditations), tactile (soft textures, temperature changes, physical movement), olfactory (essential oils, comforting scents, fresh air), and gustatory (herbal tea, mints, comfort foods in moderation).

Develop options for different settings and time constraints. Include techniques that can be used in public (breathing exercises, grounding through senses), at work (brief mindfulness practices, calming music through headphones), and at home (baths, movement, creative activities).

Test techniques during calm periods to identify what works best for your nervous system. What soothes one person might agitate another—self-soothing is highly individual and requires experimentation.

Create emergency kits for difficult situations: a playlist for your phone, essential oil roller for your purse, stress ball for your desk, and photos that bring comfort. Having tools readily available increases the likelihood you'll use them when needed.

Practice self-soothing regularly, not just during crises. Building these skills during calm moments makes them more accessible during emotional storms.

Exercise 50: Distress Tolerance Skills

Managing Overwhelming Emotions

Distress tolerance involves surviving emotional crises without making them worse through impulsive or self-destructive behaviors. These skills help you ride out intense emotional waves when soothing isn't possible or sufficient[42]. Sometimes emotions need to be experienced fully before they can resolve, and distress tolerance provides tools for enduring difficult feelings without being overwhelmed by them.

The goal isn't eliminating distress but building your capacity to handle emotional intensity without losing your grounding or engaging in behaviors that create additional problems. These skills are particularly important during schema activation when emotions feel disproportionate to current circumstances.

Case Example: Jennifer's Abandonment Crisis Management

Jennifer, a 28-year-old teacher, experienced intense emotional crises whenever her Abandonment schema was triggered. During these episodes, she would engage in behaviors that often made situations worse: calling her boyfriend repeatedly, showing up at his workplace, or threatening to end the relationship before he could leave her. Learning distress tolerance skills helped her manage these intense feelings without damaging her relationships.

126

Jennifer's distress tolerance toolkit included several specific techniques:

Temperature regulation: During panic episodes, Jennifer learned to hold ice cubes or splash cold water on her face to activate her body's diving response and slow her heart rate. This biological intervention helped interrupt the panic cycle and created space for more conscious responses.

Distraction techniques: When rumination about abandonment became overwhelming, Jennifer practiced the 5-4-3-2-1 grounding technique—identifying 5 things she could see, 4 things she could touch, 3 things she could hear, 2 things she could smell, and 1 thing she could taste. This redirected her attention from internal distress to external reality.

Radical acceptance: Jennifer practiced accepting her feelings without trying to change them immediately. She would tell herself: "This feeling is incredibly painful, and I can survive it. It will pass, just like all emotions pass. I don't have to like it or want it, but I can endure it."

Safe expression: Instead of calling her boyfriend during crises, Jennifer wrote letters expressing all her fears and feelings, then decided later if any of the content needed to be shared. This provided emotional release without creating relationship drama.

Crisis delay: Jennifer committed to waiting 24 hours before taking any major action during emotional crises. This simple rule prevented many impulsive decisions that she would later regret.

These skills helped Jennifer maintain her relationships while building confidence in her ability to handle emotional intensity. Over time, her abandonment crises became less frequent and less severe as she developed trust in her own emotional resilience.

Distress Tolerance Skill Development

Learn biological interventions that can interrupt severe emotional activation: cold water, ice cubes, intense exercise, or controlled breathing techniques. These work by engaging your body's natural regulatory systems.

Develop distraction strategies that require active engagement: complex mental tasks, physical activities, or creative projects. Passive distractions like watching TV are less effective than activities that require focus and energy.

Practice radical acceptance statements that acknowledge reality without demanding that it be different. "This is really difficult, and I can handle it" works better than "This shouldn't be happening" or "I can't stand this."

Create crisis action plans that specify what you will and won't do during emotional emergencies. Having predetermined guidelines helps you make better decisions when your thinking is clouded by intense emotions.

Build your tolerance gradually by practicing with smaller distresses before trying to use these skills during major crises. Like physical exercise, emotional tolerance improves with training.

Exercise 51: Emotion Regulation Diary

Tracking Emotional Patterns and Triggers

The Emotion Regulation Diary creates systematic awareness of your emotional patterns, triggers, and responses over time. This tracking reveals connections between external events, internal experiences, and emotional reactions that might not be obvious during single incidents. Understanding these patterns provides the foundation for targeted interventions and gradual improvement in emotional management.

Emotional tracking serves multiple purposes: it increases awareness of subtle triggers, reveals the effectiveness of different coping strategies, identifies patterns that predict difficult periods, and provides objective data about progress over time. Many people are surprised to discover how much their emotional patterns follow predictable cycles.

Case Example: David's Anger Pattern Discovery

David, a 41-year-old sales manager, kept an emotion regulation diary to understand his seemingly random episodes of intense anger that were affecting his work relationships. Initially, he believed his anger was unpredictable and uncontrollable, but the diary revealed clear patterns that allowed for targeted intervention.

David's diary entries over six weeks showed several important patterns:

Weekly cycles: His anger episodes were most frequent on Monday mornings and Friday afternoons, suggesting that work transitions and accumulated stress played significant roles in his emotional volatility.

Sleep correlation: Anger episodes were three times more likely to occur after nights when he slept fewer than six hours, indicating that fatigue was a major vulnerability factor for emotional dysregulation.

Interpersonal triggers: Specific types of interactions consistently preceded anger episodes—being interrupted during presentations, receiving last-minute requests from supervisors, and dealing with colleagues who didn't follow through on commitments.

Schema connections: The diary revealed that anger often followed situations that triggered his Defectiveness schema—moments when he felt criticized, overlooked, or treated as incompetent. The anger served as protection against underlying feelings of inadequacy and shame.

Escalation patterns: Anger episodes typically started with mild irritation that escalated over 2-3 hours if left unaddressed. Early intervention during the irritation phase was much more effective than trying to manage full-blown anger episodes.

Armed with this information, David developed targeted strategies: improving his sleep hygiene, scheduling buffer time around work transitions, practicing assertive communication to address interpersonal triggers early, and using self-soothing techniques during the irritation phase before anger escalated.

Diary Implementation Structure

Track emotions at least three times daily (morning, afternoon, evening) to capture patterns and changes throughout the day. Rate emotional intensity on a scale of 1-10 for accuracy and comparison over time.

Include both obvious emotions (anger, sadness, anxiety) and subtle ones (irritation, loneliness, restlessness). Sometimes low-level emotions provide more useful information than dramatic ones.

Note potential triggers for each emotional reaction: external events, interpersonal interactions, physical factors (sleep, hunger, illness), and internal experiences (thoughts, memories, physical sensations).

Record what you did in response to emotions and how effective those responses were. This builds awareness of which coping strategies work best for different types of emotional activation.

Look for patterns across days, weeks, and months. Are certain times particularly challenging? Do emotions follow predictable cycles? What factors seem to protect against emotional difficulties?

Exercise 52: Mindfulness for Schema Work

Present-Moment Awareness Exercises

Mindfulness provides essential skills for schema work by creating space between triggering events and automatic responses. When schemas are activated, you tend to react from past experiences rather than present realities. Mindfulness practices help you stay grounded in current circumstances while observing schema patterns without being overwhelmed by them[43].

Schema-focused mindfulness differs from general mindfulness practice by specifically targeting the patterns and reactions that maintain schema activation. These exercises help you recognize when you're being pulled into schema states and provide tools for returning to present-moment awareness where choice and flexibility are possible.

Case Example: Lisa's Perfectionism Mindfulness Practice

Lisa, a 36-year-old architect, developed mindfulness practices specifically designed to interrupt her Unrelenting Standards schema before it created overwhelming anxiety and compulsive overwork. Her mindfulness work focused on recognizing the early signs of perfectionist activation and creating space for more balanced responses.

Lisa's morning mindfulness routine included a 10-minute body scan that helped her notice physical tension that often preceded perfectionist episodes. She learned to recognize the tight feeling in her chest, shallow breathing, and clenched jaw that signaled her schema was becoming activated before her thoughts became obsessive.

During work, Lisa practiced "mindful transitions" between tasks— taking three conscious breaths and setting intentions before starting new projects. This helped her approach work from her Healthy Adult mode rather than automatically engaging her perfectionist patterns.

Lisa developed a specific mindfulness technique for handling mistakes or criticism—the STOP practice. When she noticed perfectionist thoughts arising (like "This isn't good enough" or "Everyone will think I'm incompetent"), she would:

- **S**top what she was doing
- **T**ake three deep breaths
- **O**bserve what she was thinking and feeling without judgment
- **P**roceed with conscious awareness of her choices

131

This practice helped Lisa recognize that perfectionist thoughts were just mental events, not commands that required immediate action. She could notice the thoughts, acknowledge the underlying fears, and choose how to respond based on current reality rather than schema-driven assumptions.

Lisa also practiced loving-kindness meditation specifically for her perfectionist part, sending compassion to the part of herself that worked so hard to avoid criticism and failure. This self-compassion work reduced the shame that often fueled her perfectionist cycles.

Mindfulness Practice Development

Start with brief practices (5-10 minutes) that you can maintain consistently rather than longer sessions that become burdensome. Consistency matters more than duration for building mindfulness skills.

Focus on observing schema activation without trying to stop or change it immediately. The goal is awareness and choice, not immediate elimination of schema patterns.

Practice mindfulness during neutral or positive moments, not just during crises. Building the skill during calm periods makes it more accessible during emotional storms.

Use mindfulness to observe the space between trigger and response. Even a few seconds of conscious awareness can create opportunities for different choices.

Develop specific mindfulness techniques for your most common schema patterns. Different schemas may require different approaches to mindful awareness.

Exercise 53: Self-Compassion Practices

Developing Kindness Toward Oneself

Self-compassion involves treating yourself with the same kindness you would offer a good friend facing similar difficulties. For people with schemas, self-criticism often feels more familiar and "realistic" than self-kindness, but this harsh internal treatment perpetuates the very patterns that create suffering[44]. Self-compassion practices help you develop a more nurturing internal relationship that supports healing rather than reinforcing wounds.

Self-compassion includes three components: mindfulness (awareness of suffering without being overwhelmed by it), common humanity (recognizing that struggle is part of human experience, not personal failing), and self-kindness (offering yourself warmth and understanding rather than criticism and judgment).

Case Example: Robert's Shame Healing Journey

Robert, a 43-year-old consultant, struggled with intense shame related to his Defectiveness schema. His internal voice was consistently harsh and critical, treating every mistake as evidence of his fundamental inadequacy. Self-compassion practices helped him develop a kinder, more balanced internal relationship that supported his healing work.

Robert's self-compassion practice began with learning to recognize his self-critical voice and the pain it created. He started noticing when he called himself names ("You're so stupid"), made catastrophic predictions ("You'll never succeed at anything"), or compared himself unfavorably to others ("Everyone else has their life together").

Robert developed a specific self-compassion phrase to use when shame was activated: "This is really painful right now, and I'm not the only person who feels this way. May I be kind to myself in this moment." This simple practice helped him remember that shame was a temporary experience, not a permanent truth about his worth.

Robert practiced writing self-compassionate letters to himself during difficult periods, imagining how a wise, loving friend might respond to his struggles. These letters helped him access perspectives that his shame-based thinking blocked, offering encouragement and realistic assessments of his challenges.

133

Robert also developed physical self-compassion practices: placing his hand on his heart during difficult moments, giving himself gentle hugs, and speaking to himself in the soft, warm tone he would use with a hurt child. These physical practices helped soothe his nervous system while reinforcing self-kindness.

Over time, Robert's self-compassion practice gradually replaced his automatic self-criticism with more balanced and supportive internal dialogue. He still noticed mistakes and areas for improvement, but he could address them without the intense shame that previously paralyzed him.

Self-Compassion Development Framework

Learn to recognize your self-critical voice and the specific language it uses. Does it use harsh words, absolute statements, or comparisons to others? Awareness is the first step toward change.

Develop standard self-compassion phrases that you can use during difficult moments. Having prepared responses makes it easier to access kindness when you're emotionally activated.

Practice self-compassion during small difficulties before trying to use it during major crises. Build the skill with minor frustrations, mistakes, or disappointments.

Include physical components in your self-compassion practice. Gentle touch, warm embraces, and soothing movements can activate your nervous system's caregiving responses.

Apply self-compassion specifically to your schemas and healing process. Treat your wounds and patterns with understanding rather than criticism for having them in the first place.

Exercise 54: Grounding Techniques for Dissociation

Staying Connected During Emotional Work

Dissociation represents your nervous system's attempt to protect you from overwhelming experiences by creating distance from thoughts, feelings, or bodily sensations. While this can be adaptive during trauma, chronic dissociation interferes with healing by preventing the emotional processing necessary for schema work[45]. Grounding techniques help you stay present and connected to your body and environment during difficult emotional experiences.

Effective grounding engages your senses and nervous system to maintain connection to present reality while processing challenging material. These techniques work by activating your body's natural regulatory systems and providing anchors to current experience when memories or emotions threaten to overwhelm your capacity to stay present.

Case Example: Emma's Trauma Processing Support

Emma, a 32-year-old therapist, experienced dissociation during schema work related to childhood sexual abuse. Her Detached Protector mode would automatically activate during emotional processing, leaving her feeling spacey, disconnected, and unable to access or integrate her experiences. Grounding techniques helped her stay present enough to process trauma while maintaining emotional safety.

Emma's grounding toolkit included several categories of techniques:

Sensory grounding: Emma kept a small bag of items with distinct textures, scents, and temperatures: a smooth stone, rough sandpaper, peppermint oil, and a small ice pack. During dissociative episodes, she would engage with these items to reconnect with her body and present environment.

Movement grounding: Emma practiced gentle movements that required coordination and attention: slow stretching, walking while counting steps, or simple dance movements to music. These activities helped her reconnect with her body while avoiding overwhelming intensity.

Cognitive grounding: Emma used mental exercises that required present-moment focus: naming items in her immediate environment, reciting personal information (name, age, location, date), or doing simple math problems. These activities engaged her thinking mind while staying connected to current reality.

Interpersonal grounding: Emma maintained eye contact with her therapist during difficult processing and asked for verbal anchoring ("Emma, you're here with me in my office. It's 2:30 on Tuesday afternoon. You're safe now"). This human connection helped her nervous system remain regulated during intense work.

Breathing grounding: Emma practiced specific breathing patterns that activated her parasympathetic nervous system: four counts in, hold for four, four counts out, hold for four. This rhythmic breathing provided both grounding and calming effects.

These grounding techniques allowed Emma to stay present enough for healing work while maintaining emotional safety. She could process traumatic material without losing connection to current reality and her adult resources.

Grounding Technique Development

Practice grounding during calm periods to build familiarity and effectiveness. These skills need to be well-established before being used during emotional intensity.

Engage multiple senses in your grounding practice. The more senses involved, the stronger the connection to present reality.

Keep grounding tools easily accessible. Having items readily available increases the likelihood you'll use them when needed.

Develop grounding techniques that work in different settings. Include options for public spaces, work environments, and home situations.

Combine grounding with safety statements that remind you of your current resources and supports. "I am safe now. I am an adult with choices and support. This feeling will pass."

Finding Stability in the Storm

Emotion regulation skills represent the foundation for all other schema healing work. Without the ability to manage emotional intensity, schema activation can feel overwhelming and dangerous, leading to avoidance of the very experiences needed for growth and healing. These tools provide ways to experience emotions fully while maintaining your grounding and capacity for conscious choice.

The goal isn't emotional numbing or constant calm—emotions provide essential information about your needs, values, and experiences. Instead, emotion regulation helps you develop a mature relationship with your emotional life where feelings can be experienced, expressed, and used wisely without controlling your behavior or overwhelming your capacity to function.

Building these skills requires patience and consistent practice. Your nervous system learned its current patterns over years or decades, and developing new responses takes time and repetition. Each time you practice self-soothing, use grounding techniques, or respond to emotional activation with mindfulness and self-compassion, you're creating new neural pathways that support emotional resilience and flexibility.

Success in emotion regulation often creates positive spirals that support all areas of schema healing. As you become more confident in your ability to handle emotional intensity, you become more willing to engage in challenging therapeutic work, honest self-reflection, and authentic relationships. This increased emotional courage creates opportunities for experiences that contradict schema patterns and support continued growth.

Core Elements for Emotional Freedom

- Emotional needs assessment identifies which universal needs require attention to reduce schema activation
- Self-soothing techniques provide immediate comfort during emotional distress while building regulatory capacity
- Distress tolerance skills help you survive emotional crises without making them worse through impulsive actions
- Emotion regulation diaries reveal patterns and triggers that allow for targeted intervention and prevention
- Mindfulness practices create space between schema activation and automatic responses for conscious choice
- Self-compassion work replaces harsh self-criticism with kindness and understanding that supports healing
- Grounding techniques prevent dissociation during emotional work while maintaining connection to present safety
- Regular practice builds emotional resilience and flexibility that supports all areas of personal growth

Chapter 9: Relationship and Interpersonal Exercises

Relationships serve as both the wound and the medicine in schema healing work. Your earliest relationships shaped the fundamental beliefs you carry about yourself, others, and the possibility of connection. These same beliefs now influence every interaction you have, often creating the very problems they were designed to prevent. The exercises in this section address relationship schemas directly, providing tools for recognizing interpersonal patterns and developing healthier ways of connecting with others.

Schema work in relationships requires courage because it involves risking the very things your schemas warn against—vulnerability, authenticity, and emotional intimacy. Your Abandonment schema might insist that getting close to people leads to inevitable rejection. Your Mistrust schema might argue that opening up to others invites manipulation and harm. Yet healing often requires taking these risks in small, manageable steps that gradually build evidence for new possibilities[46].

The relationship exercises in this collection recognize that interpersonal healing happens through experience, not just understanding. You can intellectually grasp that your trust issues stem from childhood betrayal, but changing those patterns requires new experiences of trustworthy relationships. These tools provide structured approaches to creating those corrective experiences while honoring your need for emotional safety.

Exercise 55: Relationship Pattern Analysis

Identifying Interpersonal Schemas

Relationship patterns often operate outside conscious awareness, creating repetitive cycles that feel like fate rather than choice. The Relationship Pattern Analysis helps you recognize these unconscious patterns by examining your history of friendships, romantic relationships, family dynamics, and professional connections. This systematic review reveals how schemas create predictable relationship outcomes across different contexts and time periods.

Effective pattern analysis looks beyond surface behaviors to identify the underlying beliefs, fears, and needs that drive interpersonal choices. You might notice that you repeatedly choose emotionally unavailable partners, struggle with the same conflicts in multiple friendships, or find yourself in similar power dynamics across different work environments. These patterns provide valuable information about which schemas require attention in relationship healing work.

Case Example: Michelle's People-Pleasing Cycle

Michelle, a 29-year-old social worker, completed a relationship pattern analysis that revealed consistent patterns across all her interpersonal connections. Her Self-Sacrifice and Subjugation schemas created cycles where she attracted people who needed help, over-gave in those relationships, became resentful when her needs weren't met, and eventually ended the relationships feeling used and exhausted.

Michelle's romantic relationships followed a predictable pattern: she would meet someone who was going through a difficult period (recent breakup, job loss, family crisis), offer extensive support and understanding, become the primary emotional caregiver in the relationship, gradually realize her partner wasn't reciprocating the same level of care, feel angry and resentful but unable to express these feelings directly, and eventually end the relationship through passive-aggressive behavior or simply withdrawing.

Her friendships showed similar patterns: Michelle was always the one people called during crises, she rarely asked for support herself, she prioritized others' needs over her own plans, she felt taken for granted but continued giving anyway, and she often felt lonely despite being surrounded by people who "needed" her.

140

Professional relationships revealed the same dynamics: Michelle volunteered for extra responsibilities, stayed late to help colleagues, took on the most difficult cases, felt overwhelmed and under-appreciated, but continued the pattern because saying no felt selfish and dangerous.

The analysis helped Michelle recognize that her schemas were creating these patterns unconsciously. Her belief that she needed to earn love through service (Self-Sacrifice) combined with her fear that expressing her own needs would lead to rejection (Subjugation) created relationships where she was valued for what she gave rather than who she was.

Michelle used this awareness to develop specific strategies for breaking her pattern: practicing expressing her needs in small ways, choosing to spend time with people who showed genuine interest in her wellbeing, setting limits on how much support she offered to others, and learning to receive care and attention without feeling obligated to reciprocate immediately.

Pattern Analysis Framework

Review your relationship history systematically across different types of connections: romantic partnerships, friendships, family relationships, and professional connections. Look for themes that appear across multiple relationships and contexts.

Identify your typical relationship roles: are you usually the caregiver, the one who needs help, the entertainer, the problem-solver, the rebel, or the peacemaker? Notice if you tend to play the same role regardless of the specific people involved.

Examine your attraction patterns: what initially draws you to people? Do you consistently choose partners with similar characteristics, problems, or relationship styles? What do you tend to overlook or dismiss in early relationship stages?

Track relationship endings: do your relationships tend to end in similar ways? Are there recurring conflicts, complaints, or issues that appear across multiple connections? What role do you typically play in relationship deterioration?

Notice your relationship fears and protective strategies: what do you worry will happen if you're truly authentic in relationships? How do you try to prevent these feared outcomes? Do these protective strategies actually create the problems you're trying to avoid?

Exercise 56: Attachment Style Assessment

Understanding Relationship Patterns

Your attachment style represents the fundamental template for how you approach relationships, developed from your earliest experiences with caregivers and refined through subsequent important relationships[47]. Understanding your attachment patterns provides essential information about your relationship schemas and guides interventions for developing more secure connections with others.

Attachment styles fall into four main categories: secure (comfortable with intimacy and autonomy), anxious (craves closeness but fears abandonment), avoidant (values independence but struggles with intimacy), and disorganized (inconsistent patterns that combine anxious and avoidant strategies). Most people with significant schemas show insecure attachment patterns that create relationship difficulties.

Case Example: James's Avoidant Attachment Recognition

James, a 35-year-old engineer, completed an attachment assessment that revealed a predominantly avoidant attachment style. His pattern involved becoming interested in relationships initially, but gradually withdrawing emotional availability as relationships became more intimate. This pattern had ended three serious relationships and was creating problems in his current partnership.

James's avoidant attachment manifested in several specific ways: he felt uncomfortable when partners expressed strong emotions, he preferred spending time alone to recharge rather than seeking comfort from others, he interpreted partners' needs for closeness as clingy or needy, he avoided discussing future plans or commitments, and he tended to minimize the importance of relationships when they became challenging.

The assessment helped James understand that his attachment style developed from childhood experiences with parents who were emotionally unavailable and critical of emotional expression. Young James learned that emotional needs were burdens and that independence was safer than dependence on others. This created an Emotional Deprivation schema that expected others to be unable or unwilling to meet his emotional needs.

Understanding his attachment pattern helped James recognize that his withdrawal wasn't a character flaw but a protective strategy that had outlived its usefulness. His current partner was emotionally available and consistently loving, but his attachment system was still operating as if emotional closeness was dangerous.

James worked on developing more secure attachment behaviors: practicing staying present during emotional conversations instead of shutting down, expressing his own needs and feelings more directly, asking for support during stressful periods instead of isolating, and responding to his partner's bids for connection with attention rather than dismissal.

The work was challenging because it required James to risk the vulnerability his attachment system was designed to avoid. However, as he practiced these new behaviors gradually, he discovered that emotional intimacy could be safe and satisfying rather than threatening and overwhelming.

Attachment Assessment Process

Evaluate your comfort with emotional intimacy: do you find it easy or difficult to get close to others? What happens to your comfort level as relationships become more intimate and committed?

Assess your response to relationship conflict: do you tend to pursue resolution actively, withdraw and shut down, become overwhelmed and emotional, or switch between different strategies inconsistently?

Examine your beliefs about relationships: do you generally trust that others will be there for you? Do you believe that people you care about will stay committed during difficult periods? Do you expect relationships to meet your emotional needs?

Notice your behavior during relationship stress: do you seek more connection or more space when relationships become challenging? How do you handle your partner's emotional distress or need for support?

Review your relationship history for patterns: do you tend to choose partners with similar attachment styles? Do your relationships end for similar reasons? Are there recurring themes in relationship conflicts or dissatisfaction?

Exercise 57: Communication Style Inventory

Recognizing Interaction Patterns

Your communication style represents how your schemas express themselves in daily interactions with others. This includes not just what you say, but how you say it, what you avoid saying, and how you interpret others' communications. Schema-driven communication often creates misunderstandings and conflicts that reinforce the very beliefs the schemas are trying to protect against.

Effective communication inventory examines both verbal and nonverbal patterns: tone of voice, body language, timing of communications, topics you avoid or emphasize, and your typical responses to different types of interpersonal situations. This awareness creates opportunities for conscious choice about how to express yourself and interpret others' messages.

Case Example: Patricia's Indirect Communication Pattern

Patricia, a 38-year-old teacher, discovered through communication inventory that her Subjugation and Approval-Seeking schemas created an indirect communication style that frequently led to misunderstandings and unmet needs. She rarely expressed disagreement directly, asked for what she needed indirectly through hints and suggestions, and interpreted others' straightforward communication as criticism or rejection.

Patricia's indirect communication manifested in several specific patterns: instead of saying no to requests, she would agree but show displeasure through sighs or delayed compliance; when she needed help, she would complain about being overwhelmed rather than asking directly; during conflicts, she would become silent or change the subject rather than addressing disagreements; and she often assumed others could read her mind about her needs and feelings.

This communication style created problems in both personal and professional relationships. Her husband felt confused by her indirect messages and frustrated by her apparent inability to tell him what she wanted. Her colleagues found her difficult to work with because she seemed agreeable in meetings but didn't follow through on commitments she'd made reluctantly.

The inventory helped Patricia recognize that her indirect style was a protective strategy designed to avoid the rejection and conflict she feared would result from direct communication. However, this protection was actually creating the relationship problems and misunderstandings she was trying to prevent.

Patricia practiced developing more direct communication skills: stating her preferences clearly instead of hoping others would guess, expressing disagreement respectfully but directly, asking for what she needed explicitly rather than hoping others would offer, and checking her interpretations of others' communications instead of assuming negative intentions.

The work required Patricia to gradually build tolerance for the anxiety that direct communication initially created. She started with low-stakes situations and practiced with people who felt safer before gradually expanding to more challenging contexts.

Communication Style Assessment

Record your typical communication patterns across different types of situations: asking for help, expressing disagreement, sharing personal information, responding to criticism, and dealing with conflict. Notice if your style changes depending on the person or context.

Identify your communication avoidance patterns: what topics do you tend to avoid? What feelings are difficult for you to express directly? What requests feel too risky to make explicitly?

Examine your nonverbal communication: what messages do you send through body language, tone of voice, and facial expressions? Do your nonverbal signals match your verbal messages?

Assess your listening patterns: do you tend to interrupt, plan your response while others are talking, or focus more on emotional tone than actual content? How do you typically respond when others share problems or feelings?

Notice your interpretation style: do you tend to assume positive or negative intentions behind others' communications? Do you take things personally that might not be about you? Do you ask for clarification when messages are unclear?

Exercise 58: Intimacy Building Exercises

Developing Closer Connections

Intimacy involves emotional closeness, vulnerability, and authentic sharing that allows others to know you deeply and accept you fully. For people with relationship schemas, intimacy often feels simultaneously desired and terrifying—you crave the connection but fear the vulnerability required to create it. Intimacy building exercises provide structured approaches to gradually increasing emotional closeness while managing the anxiety this process can create.

True intimacy requires both emotional risk-taking and boundary setting. You need to share authentic thoughts and feelings while also maintaining your individual identity and personal limits. This balance allows for genuine connection without losing yourself in relationships or pushing others away through emotional distance.

Case Example: Kevin's Gradual Vulnerability Practice

Kevin, a 31-year-old graphic designer, struggled with intimacy due to his Defectiveness and Mistrust schemas. He desperately wanted close relationships but feared that anyone who really knew him would discover his flaws and reject him. His relationships remained surface-level because he couldn't risk the vulnerability required for deeper connection.

Kevin's intimacy building plan involved gradual increases in emotional sharing and vulnerability:

Level 1 - Surface personal sharing: Kevin practiced sharing preferences, opinions, and experiences that felt relatively safe. He told friends about his favorite movies, his opinions on current events, and stories from his childhood that didn't involve emotional content.

Level 2 - Emotional reactions: Kevin began sharing his emotional responses to current events, movies, or mutual experiences. He expressed excitement about projects, disappointment about setbacks, and appreciation for friends' actions.

Level 3 - Personal struggles: Kevin started sharing current challenges he was facing: work stress, family difficulties, or personal goals he was working toward. This level required trusting that others would respond with support rather than judgment.

Level 4 - Vulnerable feelings: Kevin practiced expressing feelings that felt more risky: loneliness, insecurity, fear, or need for support.

This level directly challenged his belief that showing weakness would lead to rejection.

Level 5 - Core fears and hopes: Kevin gradually shared his deepest fears about relationships, his hopes for the future, and his most meaningful values and dreams. This level required significant trust and emotional courage.

Kevin practiced each level with different people based on the safety and trust he felt in various relationships. He started with lower levels in newer relationships while practicing higher levels with trusted friends and family members.

As Kevin practiced vulnerability gradually, he discovered that most people responded with increased warmth and openness rather than the rejection he feared. His relationships became more satisfying and supportive as he allowed others to know him more authentically.

Intimacy Building Structure

Start with relationships that already feel relatively safe and trustworthy rather than trying to build intimacy with everyone simultaneously. Success in safer relationships builds confidence for taking risks in more challenging connections.

Practice vulnerability gradually rather than sharing your deepest secrets immediately. Allow intimacy to develop naturally over time as trust and safety increase.

Balance sharing with listening: intimacy involves mutual vulnerability and support rather than one-sided emotional dumping. Ask questions about others' experiences and respond with empathy and interest.

Set appropriate boundaries while being vulnerable: you can share authentically while still maintaining privacy about topics that feel too personal or risky for particular relationships.

Pay attention to others' responses to your vulnerability: healthy relationships will respond to emotional sharing with empathy, support, and often reciprocal vulnerability. Relationships that respond with judgment, criticism, or emotional distance may not be safe for deeper intimacy.

Exercise 59: Conflict Resolution Scripts

Healthy Ways to Handle Disagreements

Conflict represents one of the greatest challenges for people with relationship schemas because it activates fears of abandonment, rejection, criticism, and harm. Many schema-driven relationship patterns involve either avoiding conflict entirely (which prevents resolution and builds resentment) or engaging in conflict destructively (which damages relationships and confirms fears about interpersonal danger). Healthy conflict resolution provides tools for addressing disagreements constructively while maintaining relationship connection.

Effective conflict resolution scripts provide specific language and approaches for expressing disagreement, setting boundaries, and working toward solutions that honor both people's needs. These scripts help you engage in necessary conflicts without being overwhelmed by schema activation or resorting to destructive communication patterns.

Case Example: Rachel's Conflict Transformation

Rachel, a 33-year-old nurse, avoided conflict in all her relationships due to her Abandonment and Approval-Seeking schemas. She believed that any disagreement would lead to rejection and loss of love. This avoidance created relationships where she felt voiceless and resentful, while others found her passive-aggressive and difficult to understand.

Rachel developed specific scripts for different types of conflicts:

For expressing disagreement: "I have a different perspective on this situation. I'd like to share my viewpoint and hear more about yours so we can understand each other better."

For setting boundaries: "I care about you and our relationship, and I need to let you know that this behavior doesn't work for me. Can we talk about how to handle this differently?"

For addressing hurt feelings: "I felt hurt when [specific behavior] happened. I don't think you intended to hurt me, but I'd like to talk about how we can prevent this in the future."

For requesting changes: "Our current approach to [specific issue] isn't working well for me. I'd like to brainstorm some alternatives that might work better for both of us."

For repair after conflict: "I know our conversation earlier was difficult. I want you to know that I value our relationship and hope we can work through this together."

Rachel practiced these scripts first with low-stakes conflicts before gradually applying them to more significant disagreements. She discovered that most people responded positively to her direct but respectful approach, and that addressing conflicts early actually strengthened her relationships rather than damaging them.

The scripts helped Rachel feel more confident during conflicts because she had specific language to use instead of either shutting down or becoming emotional. Over time, she developed her own variations that felt natural while maintaining the respectful, solution-focused approach.

Conflict Resolution Development

Identify your current conflict patterns: do you tend to avoid, attack, become emotional, shut down, or switch between different strategies? Understanding your default patterns helps you recognize when scripts might be helpful.

Practice scripts during calm periods before trying to use them during actual conflicts. Role-playing with friends or writing out potential conversations helps build familiarity and confidence.

Focus on specific behaviors rather than character attacks: "When you interrupt me during conversations" is more helpful than "You're a selfish person who doesn't care about others."

Use "I" statements to express your experience rather than "you" statements that sound like accusations: "I feel unheard" works better than "You never listen to me."

Include repair and reconnection in your conflict approach: acknowledge when conversations are difficult, express appreciation for the other person's willingness to work through issues, and actively work to rebuild connection after disagreements.

Exercise 60: Trust Building Activities

Addressing Mistrust and Abuse Schemas

Trust represents one of the most challenging areas for people with trauma histories and relationship schemas. Your Mistrust/Abuse schema may insist that everyone will eventually hurt, disappoint, or take advantage of you if given the opportunity. While this vigilance may have protected you from harm in the past, excessive mistrust can prevent you from forming the close relationships necessary for healing and happiness[48].

Trust building involves gradually testing your ability to rely on others in small ways before risking greater vulnerability. This process requires carefully chosen relationships with people who demonstrate consistent reliability, honesty, and care over time. The goal isn't naive trust of everyone, but the ability to recognize and respond appropriately to trustworthy behavior.

Case Example: Michael's Trust Rebuilding Process

Michael, a 44-year-old contractor, developed severe trust issues after childhood abuse and several adult relationships where partners betrayed his confidence or took advantage of his generosity. His Mistrust schema created hypervigilance about others' motivations and an expectation that people would eventually show their "true colors" by harming him.

Michael's trust building process involved systematic testing of trustworthiness in existing relationships:

Small reliability tests: Michael began noticing whether people followed through on minor commitments—arriving on time, returning phone calls, keeping casual promises. He practiced asking for small favors and observing whether others honored these requests.

Emotional safety tests: Michael shared slightly more personal information and observed how others responded. Did they respect his privacy, respond with empathy, or use the information against him later?

Boundary respect tests: Michael set small boundaries and noticed whether others respected them. When he said he couldn't talk on the phone after 9 PM, did others honor this limit or pressure him to make exceptions?

Consistency observation: Michael tracked whether people's behavior remained stable over time or if they showed significant mood swings, personality changes, or unpredictable responses to stress.

Reciprocity assessment: Michael observed whether relationships involved mutual care and support or if the giving was one-sided. Did others offer help when he needed it, or only seek support for themselves?

Through this systematic approach, Michael identified several relationships that consistently demonstrated trustworthy behavior over extended periods. He gradually increased his emotional investment in these relationships while maintaining appropriate caution with people who hadn't earned trust through consistent action.

Michael also worked on distinguishing between reasonable caution and schema-driven hypervigilance. His healing involved learning to trust appropriately rather than either trusting blindly or trusting no one.

Trust Building Framework

Start with small tests of reliability before risking significant vulnerability. Can this person keep minor commitments, maintain confidentiality about small matters, and respond respectfully to boundaries?

Observe behavior patterns over time rather than making trust decisions based on single interactions. Trustworthiness reveals itself through consistency across different situations and stress levels.

Notice how people handle your emotions and vulnerabilities: do they respond with empathy and respect, or do they minimize, dismiss, or use your feelings against you?

Pay attention to how others treat people with less power: their behavior toward service workers, children, or people who can't benefit them often reveals character more clearly than their treatment of equals.

Build trust gradually through reciprocal vulnerability: share something personal and observe the response before sharing something more sensitive. Healthy trust develops through mutual risk-taking over time.

Exercise 61: Relationship Boundary Worksheets

Creating Healthy Limits in Relationships

Relationship boundaries define what behavior you will and won't accept from others, what you will and won't do in relationships, and how you protect your emotional, physical, and mental wellbeing while maintaining connection with others. Poor boundaries often result from schemas that create either excessive people-pleasing (weak boundaries) or excessive withdrawal (rigid boundaries). Healthy boundaries allow for intimacy and connection while protecting your essential needs and values.

Boundary setting requires clarity about your own needs, values, and limits, as well as the communication skills to express these boundaries respectfully but firmly. This work often activates schema fears about rejection, conflict, or being seen as selfish, making it essential to develop boundaries gradually while building tolerance for others' responses.

Case Example: Sandra's Boundary Revolution

Sandra, a 36-year-old therapist, had virtually no boundaries in her personal relationships due to her Self-Sacrifice and Subjugation schemas. She allowed others to interrupt her constantly, agreed to requests she didn't want to fulfill, tolerated disrespectful behavior, and felt guilty whenever she considered her own needs. Her lack of boundaries created relationships where she felt taken advantage of and resentful.

Sandra's boundary development process involved several key areas:

Time boundaries: Sandra practiced saying no to social invitations when she needed rest, leaving parties when she felt ready rather than staying until the end, and protecting her morning routine from others' demands for immediate availability.

Emotional boundaries: Sandra learned to distinguish between empathy and emotional absorption, practicing caring about others' problems without taking responsibility for solving them. She stopped giving advice unless specifically asked and limited how much time she spent listening to others' complaints.

Physical boundaries: Sandra began expressing preferences about physical affection, personal space, and privacy. She practiced saying "I'm not comfortable with that" when others violated her physical boundaries.

154

Communication boundaries: Sandra set limits on interrupting, raised voice, and disrespectful language. She learned to say "I need you to lower your voice" or "Please let me finish speaking" when others violated these boundaries.

Financial boundaries: Sandra stopped lending money she couldn't afford to lose and began discussing financial expectations clearly in relationships. She practiced saying "That's not in my budget" without extensive explanations.

Each boundary Sandra set initially created anxiety about others' responses, but she discovered that most people respected clear, consistent limits. The few relationships that couldn't tolerate her boundaries revealed themselves to be unhealthy connections that were better ended or significantly modified.

Boundary Development Process

Identify areas where you currently lack appropriate boundaries: what behaviors do you tolerate that leave you feeling resentful, disrespected, or drained? What requests do you agree to despite not wanting to fulfill them?

Clarify your values and non-negotiables: what matters most to you in relationships? What behavior violates your core values or threatens your wellbeing?

Start with boundaries that feel important but not terrifying: build confidence with smaller limits before tackling major boundary challenges that activate intense schema fears.

Develop clear, specific language for expressing boundaries: "I need you to call before coming over" is more effective than "You need to respect my space."

Prepare for others' responses to your boundaries: some people may test limits, express disappointment, or even end relationships when you start setting boundaries. Having realistic expectations helps you maintain limits despite initial negative reactions.

Connection Through Conscious Choice

Relationship healing in schema work requires both courage and wisdom—the courage to risk vulnerability and authenticity, and the wisdom to choose relationships that can actually provide the safety and support your healing requires. The exercises in this section provide structured approaches to developing both qualities through graduated practice in real relationships.

The most powerful aspect of relationship exercises may be their ability to create new experiences that contradict schema predictions. When you practice vulnerability and receive acceptance, when you set boundaries and relationships improve, when you address conflict and connection deepens, you're gathering evidence that relationships can be different from what your schemas expect.

Success in relationship exercises often creates positive cycles that support continued growth. As your relationships become more authentic and satisfying, you gain energy and motivation for continued healing work. As you develop better relationship skills, you attract healthier partners and friends who can support your growth rather than reinforcing old patterns.

Moving Forward Together

The relationship dimension of schema healing recognizes that we are fundamentally social beings who heal through connection with others. While individual work provides essential tools and awareness, the proof of healing often shows up in your ability to form and maintain healthy, satisfying relationships that meet your needs for both connection and autonomy.

These exercises provide frameworks for creating those healthier relationships while honoring your need for emotional safety and realistic caution. The goal isn't perfect relationships or complete trust, but rather relationships that are good enough to support your growth and provide genuine satisfaction and support in daily life.

Core Principles for Relational Growth

- Relationship pattern analysis reveals how schemas create predictable interpersonal cycles across different connections
- Attachment style assessment identifies fundamental templates for approaching relationships and guides healing priorities
- Communication style awareness creates opportunities for conscious choice about how to express and interpret messages
- Intimacy building exercises provide structured approaches to increasing emotional closeness while managing vulnerability anxiety
- Conflict resolution scripts offer specific language for addressing disagreements constructively while maintaining connection
- Trust building activities help distinguish between appropriate caution and schema-driven hypervigilance
- Relationship boundary development protects wellbeing while allowing for genuine intimacy and mutual support
- Gradual practice in real relationships creates corrective experiences that contradict schema predictions about interpersonal danger

Chapter 10: Group Therapy Activities and Exercises

Group therapy provides a unique laboratory for schema healing that individual work cannot replicate. In group settings, your relationship schemas become visible through live interactions with multiple people, creating immediate opportunities to recognize patterns, practice new behaviors, and receive feedback about your interpersonal impact. The group becomes a microcosm of your broader social world, allowing you to experiment with authenticity, vulnerability, and healthy boundaries in a supportive environment[49].

The power of group work lies in its ability to provide corrective experiences that directly contradict schema predictions. Your Defectiveness schema might insist that others will reject you if they see your flaws, but group members can offer acceptance and understanding. Your Mistrust schema might warn that people will use your vulnerabilities against you, but group experiences can demonstrate genuine care and protection of shared confidences.

Group schema therapy requires careful structure and skilled facilitation to create psychological safety while encouraging the kind of authentic interaction that promotes healing. The exercises in this section provide frameworks for group work that balance individual needs with collective healing, creating experiences that benefit both individual members and the group as a whole.

Exercise 62: Group Schema Check-In

Opening Ritual for Group Sessions

The Group Schema Check-In provides a structured beginning for each group session that helps members connect with their current internal state, share their emotional reality with others, and begin building the emotional intimacy necessary for therapeutic work. This exercise creates predictable safety while allowing for spontaneous sharing that reflects each member's immediate needs and concerns.

Effective check-ins balance structure with flexibility, ensuring that everyone has opportunity to share while accommodating different comfort levels with self-disclosure. The format provides language and framework for members who might struggle with identifying or expressing their emotional states while encouraging authentic sharing rather than surface-level social pleasantries.

Case Example: Tuesday Evening Group Dynamics

The Tuesday evening schema therapy group consisted of eight members dealing with various relationship and self-worth schemas. Their check-in process had evolved over months to include both current emotional states and any schema activation they'd experienced since the previous session.

During one typical check-in, Sarah (struggling with Abandonment schema) shared: "I'm feeling anxious tonight because my boyfriend seemed distant this weekend. My abandonment schema is telling me he's losing interest, but my healthier voice recognizes he's just stressed about work deadlines. I want to work on trusting the evidence instead of my fear."

Mark (dealing with Defectiveness schema) followed: "I'm feeling frustrated with myself because I made a mistake on a project at work, and I've been beating myself up for three days. I know logically that mistakes are normal, but emotionally I feel like this proves I'm not good enough for my job. I'd like to practice some self-compassion tonight."

Jennifer (working with Self-Sacrifice schema) added: "I'm exhausted because I agreed to help my sister move this weekend even though I had planned to rest. I did it again—said yes when I wanted to say no. I'm angry at myself for not setting boundaries, and I'm hoping the group can help me figure out how to handle this differently next time."

These check-ins accomplished several therapeutic goals simultaneously: they helped members articulate their current emotional reality, connected current experiences to ongoing schema work, normalized struggles and setbacks, created opportunities for group support and feedback, and set the stage for more focused therapeutic work during the session.

The group leader used the check-ins to identify themes for the session, notice members who might need extra support, and help the group understand how individual schema work connected to collective healing.

Check-In Structure Development

Create a consistent format that includes emotional state, recent schema activation, and current needs or goals for the session. This structure helps members organize their sharing while ensuring important elements are addressed.

Encourage specific rather than general sharing: "I'm feeling anxious about a conversation with my boss" provides more useful information than "I'm fine" or "It's been a hard week."

Include both struggles and successes in check-ins: share schema activation and difficulties as well as moments of healthy response and growth. This balanced approach prevents sessions from becoming purely problem-focused.

Allow flexibility in sharing depth: some members may share extensively while others offer briefer updates. Both styles can be valuable for group learning and connection.

Use check-ins to identify session themes and priorities: patterns across multiple members' experiences often reveal important topics for group exploration.

Exercise 63: Schema Mode Role-Play

Group Exercises for Mode Work

Schema Mode Role-Play allows group members to practice recognizing and working with different modes through structured dramatic exercises. Members can play their own modes, represent modes for other group members, or practice strengthening their Healthy Adult mode through interaction with others' schema patterns. These exercises make abstract concepts concrete while providing safe practice for real-world mode management.

Mode role-play creates opportunities for group members to see their patterns from outside perspectives, receive feedback about how their modes affect others, and practice responding to different modes with compassion and skill. The group setting allows for multiple perspectives and creative solutions that individual work might not generate.

Case Example: Lisa's Demanding Parent Workshop

During a group session focused on mode work, Lisa volunteered to explore her Demanding Parent mode that created chronic stress and damaged her relationships through impossible expectations. The group designed a role-play exercise where different members represented various aspects of Lisa's internal world.

Tom played Lisa's Demanding Parent mode, sitting in a chair positioned above the others and speaking in harsh, urgent tones: "You can't relax now—there's still work to be done! If you don't stay ahead of everything, you'll fall behind and people will see that you're not as competent as they thought. You have to be perfect or you're worthless."

Sarah represented Lisa's Vulnerable Child mode, sitting small in her chair and responding with anxiety and exhaustion: "I'm so tired of trying to be perfect. Nothing I do is ever good enough for you. I just want to rest and feel okay about myself without having to achieve something constantly."

Jennifer embodied Lisa's Healthy Adult mode, standing between the other two chairs and addressing both parts with wisdom and compassion: "I hear that you're both trying to protect Lisa in your own ways. Demanding Parent, I understand you're scared of failure and criticism. Vulnerable Child, I see how exhausted you are from these impossible standards."

The Healthy Adult continued: "What if we could work together differently? We can maintain high standards for truly important things while relaxing our expectations for routine tasks. We can achieve excellence without demanding perfection. Lisa is competent and valued regardless of her performance."

The role-play allowed Lisa to see her internal conflict from an external perspective and gave the group practice in accessing their own Healthy Adult modes. Other members offered suggestions for how the Healthy Adult could mediate between the conflicting parts, and Lisa gained concrete language for internal dialogues.

Role-Play Implementation Guidelines

Choose volunteers who feel comfortable with dramatic expression while ensuring that shy members have alternative ways to participate such as offering suggestions or feedback.

Start with less intense modes before working with highly emotional or traumatic material. Build group comfort and safety through success with manageable scenarios.

Debrief thoroughly after role-plays to process emotional reactions, insights gained, and applications to real-life situations. The discussion often provides as much learning as the exercise itself.

Encourage creativity and spontaneity while maintaining respect for each member's emotional safety. Role-plays should feel playful and experimental rather than critiquing or analyzing.

Connect role-play insights to practical applications: how can group members use what they learned during the exercise in their daily lives and relationships?

Exercise 64: Peer Support Partnerships

Buddy System for Accountability

Peer Support Partnerships create structured relationships between group members that extend therapeutic support beyond group sessions. Partners check in with each other regularly, provide encouragement during difficult periods, and offer accountability for practicing new behaviors and completing therapeutic homework. These relationships model healthy interdependence while providing practical support for schema healing work.

Effective partnerships balance mutual support with individual responsibility, ensuring that both members benefit from the relationship without creating dependency or caretaking dynamics that might reinforce schema patterns. The partnerships provide opportunities to practice healthy relationship skills in a supportive context.

Case Example: David and Michael's Accountability Alliance

David (working with Emotional Inhibition schema) and Michael (addressing Social Isolation schema) formed a peer support partnership that helped both members make significant progress in their healing work. Their different schema patterns actually complemented each other's growth needs.

David struggled with expressing emotions and asking for support, while Michael avoided social connection due to fears of rejection and judgment. Their partnership provided safe practice for both members to work on their specific challenges.

Their weekly check-ins followed a structured format: each member shared their emotional state, any schema activation they'd experienced, progress on therapeutic goals, and specific support needs for the coming week. David practiced emotional expression by sharing his feelings honestly, while Michael practiced social

163

connection by initiating contact and maintaining consistent communication.

During David's particularly stressful work period, Michael offered practical support by calling daily to check in and providing a listening ear without trying to solve David's problems. This helped David practice receiving support while giving Michael experience in offering care without taking responsibility for another's wellbeing.

When Michael felt tempted to isolate after a social rejection, David provided gentle accountability by encouraging him to attend their planned group session and reminding him of previous social successes. This helped Michael resist his schema's urge to withdraw while giving David practice in supportive confrontation.

Their partnership also included practicing new behaviors together: they attended social events as a team, practiced assertive communication through role-play, and celebrated each other's progress and achievements. These shared experiences provided evidence that relationships could be supportive and growth-oriented rather than threatening or demanding.

Partnership Structure Development

Match partners based on complementary growth goals rather than similar schemas: different schema patterns can provide unique support and learning opportunities for each other.

Establish clear expectations about frequency and format of contact: weekly phone calls, text check-ins, or in-person meetings depending on members' preferences and availability.

Create structure for partnership interactions that ensures mutual benefit rather than one-sided support: both members should have opportunities to give and receive support.

Include accountability elements that feel supportive rather than controlling: partners can remind each other of goals and commitments while respecting autonomy and choice.

Plan partnership duration and evaluation: some partnerships work well short-term while others develop into lasting friendships. Regular evaluation helps ensure the relationship continues serving both members' growth.

Exercise 65: Group Imagery Exercises

Collective Visualization Activities

Group imagery exercises involve shared visualization experiences that create collective healing opportunities while addressing individual schema patterns. These exercises can include guided imagery led by the facilitator, member-led visualizations based on personal healing experiences, or collaborative imagery creation where the group builds healing scenarios together. The shared experience creates powerful bonds while providing multiple perspectives on healing possibilities.

Group imagery work often feels more powerful than individual visualization because the collective energy and shared intention amplify the healing impact. Members also benefit from hearing others' imagery experiences, which can suggest new possibilities for their own healing work.

Case Example: The Group's Safe Haven Creation

During a particularly intense group session dealing with trauma-related schemas, the facilitator led a collective imagery exercise to create a shared safe space that all members could access during difficult moments. The group collaborated to design an imaginary retreat center that incorporated elements meaningful to each member.

The imagery began with the facilitator guiding the group to a beautiful natural setting—a meadow surrounded by mountains with a clear stream running through it. Each member contributed elements to the scene: Sarah added a cozy log cabin with a fireplace, Mark included a garden with healing herbs, Jennifer placed comfortable seating areas for conversation, David contributed a library with inspiring books, and Michael added walking trails for solitary reflection.

The group spent time exploring their collective creation, with each member describing what they saw, heard, and felt in this shared sacred space. They discussed how the different elements met various healing needs: the cabin provided warmth and shelter, the garden offered beauty and growth symbolism, the seating areas enabled connection and support, the library represented wisdom and learning, and the trails honored needs for solitude and reflection.

Members agreed to visit this shared safe space during individual meditation or difficult moments, knowing that others in the group might be connecting with the same healing environment. This created a sense of ongoing connection and mutual support that extended beyond group sessions.

Several members reported accessing the shared imagery during challenging weeks and feeling comforted by the sense of connection to other group members even when physically apart. The exercise had created a portable resource that combined individual healing with group bonding.

Group Imagery Development

Choose imagery themes that address common schema concerns while allowing for individual variation: safety, nurturing, strength, wisdom, or future healing are universal needs that can be personalized.

Include both guided and collaborative elements: facilitator-led imagery provides structure while member contributions create ownership and personal meaning.

Allow time for sharing and processing imagery experiences: the discussion often provides as much healing value as the visualization itself.

Connect imagery experiences to practical applications: how can group members access these healing resources during daily life challenges?

Create ongoing imagery resources that the group can reference and build upon over time: shared safe spaces, healing figures, or strength symbols that become part of the group's collective identity.

Exercise 66: Schema Sharing Circles

Structured Disclosure Exercises

Schema Sharing Circles provide structured opportunities for group members to share their schema stories in depth while receiving support and validation from others with similar experiences. These exercises move beyond surface-level sharing to include the origins, impacts, and healing journeys associated with specific schemas. The structured format ensures psychological safety while encouraging authentic vulnerability.

Sharing circles work by normalizing schema experiences, reducing shame and isolation, providing multiple perspectives on healing possibilities, and creating deep emotional connections between group members. The format honors each person's story while building collective wisdom about schema healing.

Case Example: The Abandonment Schema Circle

During one memorable session, three group members (Sarah, Jennifer, and Tom) shared their experiences with Abandonment schemas in a structured circle format. Each member had 15 minutes to share their story while others listened without interruption, followed by 10 minutes of supportive response and questions.

Sarah shared first, describing how her father's sudden departure when she was seven created a deep belief that people she loved would inevitably leave without warning. She described the hypervigilance she experienced in relationships, constantly scanning for signs of withdrawal or loss of interest. She also shared her progress in learning to distinguish between schema fears and relationship reality.

Jennifer followed, sharing how her mother's emotional unavailability due to depression created abandonment fears focused on emotional rather than physical departure. She described feeling invisible and unimportant in relationships, constantly working to earn attention and care. Her healing work involved learning to value herself independently of others' approval.

Tom shared his abandonment story rooted in multiple foster placements during childhood, creating a belief that all relationships were temporary and that getting too attached would inevitably lead to loss. He described his tendency to end relationships preemptively to avoid being left, and his current work on allowing himself to care deeply despite uncertainty about permanence.

The sharing revealed both common themes (fear of loss, hypervigilance, relationship testing) and unique variations (physical versus emotional abandonment, different triggering events, various coping strategies). Members felt deeply understood and less alone in their struggles.

The supportive responses included validation of each person's experience, appreciation for their courage in sharing, and practical suggestions for continued healing. The circle created lasting bonds between members who felt seen and accepted despite their deepest fears and vulnerabilities.

Sharing Circle Structure

Establish clear guidelines for sharing and responding that ensure safety and respect: no interrupting during shares, no advice-giving unless requested, and confidentiality about personal details shared.

Create time limits that allow for depth while ensuring all members can participate: 10-15 minutes for sharing with 5-10 minutes for responses works well for most groups.

Choose specific themes or schemas to focus each circle rather than allowing completely open sharing: structure helps members prepare and ensures relevance for all participants.

Include both story-sharing and current healing work: historical background provides context while current efforts offer hope and practical ideas.

Follow sharing circles with integration time for processing emotions, insights, and connections to individual healing work.

Exercise 67: Group Behavioral Experiments

Collective Pattern-Breaking Activities

Group Behavioral Experiments involve the entire group participating in activities designed to challenge schema-driven avoidance and test new behavioral responses. These experiments provide safety through numbers while creating opportunities for immediate feedback and support. The group setting makes challenging behaviors feel less risky while providing multiple witnesses to successful outcomes.

Collective experiments work particularly well for addressing social schemas like Social Isolation, Approval-Seeking, or Subjugation that involve interpersonal fears and avoidance. The group provides built-in social interaction opportunities and immediate evidence about others' responses to authentic self-expression.

Case Example: The Restaurant Assertiveness Challenge

A group of six members dealing with various schemas that interfered with assertiveness decided to conduct a collective behavioral experiment at a local restaurant. The experiment was designed to challenge each member's specific avoidance patterns while providing group support and encouragement.

The experiment involved several mini-challenges tailored to individual schemas:

Sarah (Abandonment schema) practiced expressing preferences by requesting a specific table location and asking for modifications to her meal order. Her schema insisted that making requests would annoy others and lead to rejection, but the restaurant staff responded helpfully and the group provided positive feedback about her assertiveness.

Mark (Defectiveness schema) challenged his pattern of over-apologizing by resisting the urge to apologize for normal requests and needs. He practiced saying "Could I have some extra napkins?" instead of "I'm sorry to bother you, but could I possibly have some napkins if it's not too much trouble?" The group helped him notice how much more confident and appropriate his direct requests sounded.

Jennifer (Self-Sacrifice schema) practiced ordering what she actually wanted rather than choosing based on price or what she thought others expected. She ordered the slightly more expensive item she preferred instead of automatically selecting the cheapest option. The group celebrated her choice to prioritize her own preferences.

David (Emotional Inhibition schema) practiced expressing authentic reactions by commenting on the food, atmosphere, and his enjoyment of the group experience. Instead of his usual reserved responses, he shared his genuine appreciation for the restaurant's ambiance and the quality of his meal.

Michael (Social Isolation schema) practiced initiating conversation by asking the server about menu recommendations and engaging in brief small talk. His schema warned that others would find him awkward or annoying, but the interactions flowed naturally and pleasantly.

Tom (Approval-Seeking schema) practiced expressing a minority opinion when the group discussed their meals, sharing that he didn't enjoy his dish as much as others seemed to enjoy theirs. Instead of automatically agreeing with the group consensus, he expressed his authentic experience while remaining respectful of others' different preferences.

The collective experiment provided immediate evidence that challenged each member's schema predictions while creating a fun, bonding experience for the group. Members supported each other

170

through anxiety, celebrated successful challenges, and processed their experiences together afterward.

Collective Experiment Design

Choose activities that provide natural opportunities for multiple schema challenges rather than artificial or contrived situations. Real-world settings provide more meaningful evidence than role-plays.

Ensure experiments feel challenging but achievable for group members' current skill levels. Success builds confidence for future challenges while overwhelming experiences can reinforce schema beliefs.

Plan specific challenges for each member based on their individual schema patterns and avoidance behaviors. Personalized experiments provide more targeted therapeutic benefit.

Include group processing time immediately after experiments to capture fresh reactions, insights, and emotional responses before they fade from memory.

Connect experiment outcomes to ongoing therapeutic work by discussing how successful experiences can inform future behavioral choices and challenge schema predictions.

Exercise 68: Termination and Closure Rituals

Ending Group Therapy Meaningfully

Group termination requires careful attention to closure processes that honor the relationships formed, acknowledge the growth achieved, and prepare members for continued healing work outside the group context. Termination rituals help members integrate their group experience while managing the grief and anxiety that often accompany therapeutic endings.

Effective termination addresses both practical elements (sharing contact information, discussing continued therapy plans) and emotional elements (expressing appreciation, processing grief about endings, celebrating achievements). The ritual aspect provides structure for complex emotions while creating meaningful closure.

Case Example: The Tuesday Group's Graduation Ceremony

After 18 months together, the Tuesday evening schema therapy group prepared for termination with a multi-week closure process that honored their shared journey and individual growth. The group designed their own graduation ceremony that incorporated elements meaningful to their collective experience.

The ceremony began with each member sharing their most significant learning from the group experience and how they had grown during their time together. Sarah spoke about learning to trust her own perceptions instead of constantly questioning herself. Mark discussed developing self-compassion and reducing his harsh self-criticism. Jennifer shared her progress in setting boundaries and valuing her own needs.

Members exchanged written appreciations highlighting specific ways each person had contributed to others' healing. These letters addressed both personal qualities (courage, humor, wisdom) and specific moments of support or insight that had made differences in individual healing journeys.

The group created a collective timeline of their shared experience, noting significant moments, breakthroughs, challenges overcome, and funny memories that had bonded them together. This timeline became a visual representation of their collective growth and shared history.

Each member contributed to a group wisdom book containing insights, quotes, exercises, and reminders that had been meaningful during their work together. They made copies for everyone to take as ongoing resources for continued healing work.

The ceremony concluded with each member lighting a candle while stating their commitment to continued growth and healing after the group ended. The ritual provided both closure for their shared experience and launching energy for individual journeys ahead.

The group also addressed practical elements: sharing contact information for those who wanted to maintain friendships, discussing individual therapy plans, and creating agreements about confidentiality and future contact that honored both connection and appropriate boundaries.

Termination Ritual Development

Begin termination processing several weeks before the actual end to allow time for emotional processing and meaningful closure activities.

Include both individual reflection and group sharing elements that honor personal growth within the context of collective healing.

Create tangible reminders of the group experience that members can take with them: photos, letters, artwork, or written materials that capture shared wisdom and memories.

Address both celebration of growth and grief about ending: termination involves complex emotions that deserve acknowledgment and processing.

Plan for post-group contact and support in ways that honor therapeutic boundaries while allowing for appropriate ongoing connection when desired.

The Healing Power of Witnessed Change

Group therapy provides unique opportunities for schema healing that individual work cannot replicate. The group setting creates a laboratory for practicing new interpersonal behaviors, receiving immediate feedback about your impact on others, and witnessing others' courage in facing similar challenges. These shared experiences often accelerate healing by providing evidence that contradicts schema predictions about relationships and self-worth.

The exercises in this section provide structured approaches to group work that balance individual healing needs with collective growth opportunities. Each activity creates multiple learning opportunities: you benefit from your own participation, from observing others' experiences, and from the group connections that develop through shared vulnerability and support.

Perhaps most importantly, group work addresses the fundamental human need for belonging and acceptance that underlies many schemas. When group members accept you despite knowing your struggles, when they value your contributions even during difficult periods, and when they continue caring about you through setbacks and mistakes, you gain experiential evidence that relationships can be safe, supportive, and healing.

A Community of Growth

The transition from group therapy to independent living often feels daunting, but the relationships and skills developed through group work create lasting resources for continued growth. Many group members maintain friendships that provide ongoing support and accountability. Others carry the internalized voices of group members who offered encouragement and perspective during difficult times.

The group experience teaches essential lessons about healthy interdependence—the ability to give and receive support, to be both independent and connected, and to contribute to others' wellbeing while caring for your own needs. These skills transfer directly to relationships outside the therapy setting, creating ripple effects that extend the healing impact far beyond the group experience itself.

Essential Elements for Group Healing

- Group schema check-ins create predictable safety while encouraging authentic sharing about current struggles and growth
- Schema mode role-play makes abstract concepts concrete while providing safe practice for real-world mode management
- Peer support partnerships extend therapeutic support beyond group sessions through structured accountability relationships
- Group imagery exercises create collective healing experiences that amplify individual visualization work
- Schema sharing circles provide structured opportunities for deep disclosure while building connections through shared vulnerability
- Group behavioral experiments challenge avoidance patterns through collective support and immediate evidence gathering
- Termination rituals honor relationships formed while preparing members for continued independent growth
- Group experiences provide corrective relationships that contradict schema predictions about interpersonal danger and rejection

Chapter 11: Progress Tracking and Measurement Tools

Healing happens gradually, often in ways too subtle to notice day by day. You might feel like you're making no progress while actually experiencing significant positive changes that become visible only through systematic tracking over time. The exercises in this section provide objective methods for measuring therapeutic progress, identifying patterns of improvement, and maintaining motivation during the inevitable plateaus and setbacks that characterize deep healing work[51].

Progress tracking serves multiple essential functions: it provides evidence of change when subjective experience feels static, identifies which interventions produce the most benefit, reveals patterns in setbacks that suggest environmental or timing factors, and creates accountability for therapeutic goals and commitments. Without systematic measurement, clients often underestimate their progress and therapists miss important patterns that could inform treatment adjustments.

Schema healing involves changes across multiple domains— emotional regulation, relationship patterns, self-talk, behavioral choices, life satisfaction, and overall functioning. Effective progress tracking measures these different areas while remaining simple enough to maintain consistently over extended periods. The goal is creating useful information that supports continued growth rather than burdensome record-keeping that becomes another source of stress.

Exercise 69: Weekly Schema Progress Review

Regular Assessment of Changes

The Weekly Schema Progress Review provides a systematic framework for assessing changes in schema activation, coping responses, and overall functioning on a regular basis. This tool helps identify both obvious improvements and subtle shifts that might otherwise go unnoticed. Weekly tracking captures patterns that daily monitoring might miss while remaining frequent enough to provide useful feedback for treatment adjustments.

Effective weekly reviews balance comprehensiveness with practicality, measuring the most important indicators of progress without creating an overwhelming assessment burden. The review should take 10-15 minutes to complete and provide information that genuinely helps guide therapeutic decisions and personal growth efforts.

Case Example: Maria's Perfectionism Progress Journey

Maria, a 34-year-old marketing director, completed weekly schema progress reviews for six months while working on her Unrelenting Standards schema. Her systematic tracking revealed patterns of improvement that weren't obvious from her subjective experience during difficult weeks.

Maria's weekly review included several key measurements:

Schema Activation Frequency: Maria rated how often her perfectionist schema was triggered during the week on a scale of 1-10. Early reviews showed consistent scores of 8-9, but after three months, scores typically ranged from 4-6, with occasional spikes during particularly stressful periods.

Emotional Intensity: When perfectionist thoughts arose, Maria rated their emotional impact from 1-10. While the frequency of activation decreased gradually, the intensity of emotional reactions dropped more dramatically—from overwhelming anxiety that lasted hours to brief discomfort that resolved within minutes.

Coping Response Quality: Maria tracked how effectively she responded to schema activation using healthy strategies like self-compassion, realistic standards, and time boundaries. Her scores showed steady improvement as new responses became more automatic and effective.

Functional Impact: Maria measured how much her perfectionism interfered with work productivity, relationship satisfaction, and personal well-being. This metric showed the most dramatic improvement, as she learned to maintain high standards without sacrificing other life areas.

Behavioral Changes: Maria tracked specific behavioral changes like leaving work on time, saying no to non-essential tasks, and completing projects without excessive revision. These concrete behaviors provided objective evidence of progress beyond subjective feelings.

The weekly tracking revealed several important patterns: Maria's progress wasn't linear, with some weeks showing temporary increases in schema activation during stressful periods. However, the overall trend was clearly positive, and recovery from setbacks became faster over time. Most importantly, even when schema activation occurred, its impact on her functioning and relationships decreased significantly.

Review Implementation Structure

Select 5-7 key indicators that represent the most important aspects of your schema healing work: activation frequency, emotional intensity, coping effectiveness, functional impact, and specific behavioral changes.

Use consistent rating scales (typically 1-10) that allow for comparison across weeks and identification of trends over time. Brief written notes can supplement numerical ratings to provide context.

Complete reviews at the same time each week to establish routine and ensure consistency. Sunday evenings or Monday mornings work well for reflecting on the previous week and setting intentions for the week ahead.

Track both struggles and successes to maintain balanced perspective. Progress includes both reducing problematic patterns and increasing healthy responses.

Review accumulated data monthly to identify longer-term trends and patterns that weekly snapshots might miss. Look for seasonal variations, life stress correlations, and intervention effectiveness patterns.

Exercise 70: Goal Setting and Achievement Tracker

Specific, Measurable Objectives

The Goal Setting and Achievement Tracker provides a systematic approach to identifying therapeutic objectives and monitoring progress toward their completion. This tool helps translate abstract healing concepts into concrete, actionable goals that can be measured and achieved within specific timeframes. Clear goal setting increases motivation, provides direction for therapeutic work, and creates opportunities for celebrating progress.

Effective therapeutic goals balance ambition with achievability, specificity with flexibility, and individual preferences with clinical recommendations. Goals should be meaningful to the client, realistic given current circumstances, and specific enough to allow clear measurement of achievement.

Case Example: Robert's Relationship Goal Development

Robert, a 39-year-old teacher, struggled with Social Isolation and Emotional Deprivation schemas that left him feeling lonely and disconnected despite being surrounded by colleagues and acquaintances. His goal-setting process helped transform vague desires for "better relationships" into specific, achievable objectives.

Robert's six-month goals included several categories:

Social Connection Goals:

- Initiate lunch with a colleague once per month (achieved 5 out of 6 months)

- Join one social activity outside of work (joined hiking club in month 2)
- Attend at least 75% of optional work social events (achieved 80% attendance)
- Have one meaningful conversation per week (tracked and consistently achieved)

Emotional Expression Goals:

- Share one personal detail per week with trusted colleague (tracked daily, achieved 90% of weeks)
- Express appreciation to others twice per week (exceeded goal consistently)
- Ask for help or support when needed rather than struggling alone (achieved 60% improvement)
- Practice vulnerability by sharing struggles with appropriate people (achieved in 3 significant conversations)

Boundary Setting Goals:

- Say no to requests that conflict with personal time twice per month (achieved 100%)
- Limit work-related activities to 50 hours per week (achieved 80% of weeks)
- Take full lunch breaks instead of working through them (achieved 85% of workdays)
- Schedule one purely enjoyable activity per week (achieved 90% of weeks)

Communication Skills Goals:

- Practice active listening by asking follow-up questions in conversations (became automatic by month 4)
- Express disagreement respectfully when it occurs rather than staying silent (achieved in 8 situations)
- Compliment others genuinely when opportunities arise (exceeded goal significantly)
- Share opinions in group settings rather than remaining silent (achieved 70% improvement)

The tracking revealed that Robert achieved most of his goals while discovering that some objectives were too ambitious for his starting point. He learned to adjust goals based on experience while maintaining forward momentum through consistent small successes.

Goal Development Framework

Create goals that are specific, measurable, achievable, relevant, and time-bound (SMART criteria). Vague goals like "improve relationships" become specific objectives like "initiate one social conversation per week."

Include both behavioral goals (actions you can take) and outcome goals (results you want to achieve). Behavioral goals are more directly controllable while outcome goals provide motivation and direction.

Set goals across multiple life domains affected by your schemas: relationships, work, self-care, emotional regulation, and personal growth. Balanced goals prevent over-focus on single areas.

Establish both short-term goals (weekly or monthly) and longer-term objectives (quarterly or yearly). Short-term goals provide frequent success experiences while long-term goals maintain overall direction.

Build in flexibility for goal adjustment based on experience and changing circumstances. The goal-setting process should support growth rather than creating additional pressure and self-criticism.

Exercise 71: Therapy Milestone Celebrations

Recognizing Progress and Growth

Therapy Milestone Celebrations provide structured opportunities to acknowledge and celebrate significant achievements in schema healing work. These celebrations serve important psychological functions: they reinforce positive changes through recognition and reward, build motivation for continued effort, create positive

181

associations with therapeutic work, and help integrate new identity elements that reflect growth and healing.

Milestone celebrations work by making abstract progress concrete and memorable. Instead of healing feeling like an endless process with no clear achievements, milestones create specific moments of completion and success that can be remembered and referenced during difficult periods.

Case Example: Jennifer's Six-Month Transformation Recognition

Jennifer, a 31-year-old nurse, had worked intensively on her Self-Sacrifice schema for six months with significant results that deserved recognition and celebration. Her therapy milestone celebration honored both specific achievements and overall transformation.

Jennifer's milestone celebration included several elements:

Achievement Documentation: Jennifer created a written record of specific changes she'd accomplished: setting boundaries with family members about holiday obligations, saying no to overtime requests when she needed rest, asking for help with household tasks instead of doing everything herself, expressing her needs directly rather than hoping others would guess, and choosing activities based on her interests rather than others' expectations.

Before and After Comparison: Jennifer wrote letters from her "old self" to her "new self" highlighting how her daily experience had changed. The old self letter described constant exhaustion, resentment, and feeling taken for granted. The new self letter expressed appreciation for boundaries, authentic relationships, and self-respect.

Support Person Inclusion: Jennifer invited her sister and best friend to her celebration, sharing how they had supported her growth and asking them to reflect on changes they'd observed. Their feedback provided external validation of her progress and helped her see improvements she might have minimized.

Symbolic Actions: Jennifer performed symbolic actions that represented her growth: she donated clothes that represented her "people-pleasing" image, bought something special for herself without feeling guilty, and wrote a letter of appreciation to herself acknowledging her courage in changing difficult patterns.

Future Commitment: Jennifer made commitments for continued growth while celebrating current achievements. She identified areas for continued development while honoring how far she'd come.

The celebration helped Jennifer internalize her progress and feel genuinely proud of her achievements rather than immediately moving on to the next area needing improvement. This positive reinforcement supported continued motivation for therapeutic work.

Celebration Design Elements

Identify specific, concrete achievements that deserve recognition rather than celebrating vague or minimal progress. Genuine accomplishments provide more meaningful celebration opportunities.

Include both individual reflection and social recognition when possible. Support from others amplifies the positive impact of milestone acknowledgment.

Create tangible reminders of achievements that can be referenced during difficult periods: certificates, photos, letters, or objects that symbolize growth and progress.

Balance celebration of past achievements with commitment to continued growth. Milestones mark progress within an ongoing journey rather than final destinations.

Schedule regular milestone reviews to ensure progress gets recognized rather than overlooked in the focus on remaining challenges.

Exercise 72: Setback Recovery Planning

Managing Therapy Obstacles

Setback Recovery Planning acknowledges that therapeutic progress rarely follows a straight upward trajectory. Instead, healing involves cycles of progress, plateau periods, and temporary returns to old patterns that can feel discouraging and confusing. This tool helps normalize setbacks while providing specific strategies for recovering quickly and learning from temporary obstacles.

Effective setback recovery planning distinguishes between normal fluctuations in progress and more serious therapy obstacles that require professional intervention. The framework provides immediate coping strategies while helping identify patterns that might predict and prevent future setbacks.

Case Example: David's Perfectionism Relapse Navigation

David, a 41-year-old consultant, experienced a significant setback in his Unrelenting Standards schema work during a particularly stressful project deadline. After months of progress in setting realistic standards and maintaining work-life balance, he returned to 12-hour workdays, obsessive revision cycles, and harsh self-criticism that left him exhausted and demoralized.

David's setback recovery plan helped him navigate this challenge effectively:

Immediate Damage Control: David recognized the setback early and implemented immediate interventions to prevent further deterioration: he set a firm deadline for ending work each day, reached out to his therapist for an emergency session, used self-compassion exercises to counter self-criticism, and asked his partner for extra support during the stressful period.

Pattern Analysis: David analyzed what had triggered the setback and what factors had made him vulnerable: the high-stakes nature of the project activated his fear of failure, sleep deprivation had reduced his emotional regulation capacity, isolation from support systems had left him without reality-checking resources, and old workplace dynamics had triggered familiar perfectionist responses.

Learning Integration: David identified specific lessons from the setback that could prevent future occurrences: recognizing early warning signs of perfectionist activation, maintaining support connections during stressful periods, setting preemptive boundaries around work hours during high-pressure projects, and developing contingency plans for handling fear-based decision making.

Recovery Strategies: David implemented specific strategies to return to healthier patterns: he scheduled regular check-ins with his therapist during stressful periods, created accountability partnerships with colleagues who supported his boundary-setting efforts, developed written reminders of his values and priorities that he could reference during schema activation, and practiced self-forgiveness for the temporary return to old patterns.

Prevention Planning: David used the setback experience to strengthen his overall recovery by identifying vulnerability factors and developing specific prevention strategies for similar future situations.

The setback ultimately strengthened David's schema work by providing real-world practice in recovery skills and deeper understanding of his vulnerability patterns.

Recovery Planning Development

Normalize setbacks as expected parts of the healing process rather than evidence of failure or lack of progress. This perspective reduces shame and supports faster recovery.

Develop immediate intervention strategies that can be implemented quickly when setbacks occur: emergency coping skills, support contacts, and boundary-setting actions.

Include pattern analysis to understand setback triggers and vulnerability factors: stress levels, life circumstances, social support, and environmental factors that increase setback risk.

Create learning integration processes that help extract value from setback experiences: what information does this provide about your healing process and what adjustments might be helpful?

Build prevention strategies based on setback analysis: specific actions that can reduce vulnerability and early intervention approaches that prevent minor slips from becoming major relapses.

Exercise 73: Quality of Life Assessment

Measuring Overall Life Satisfaction

The Quality of Life Assessment provides a broader perspective on therapeutic progress by measuring satisfaction and functioning across multiple life domains rather than focusing solely on symptom reduction or specific therapeutic targets. This tool recognizes that the ultimate goal of schema healing is improved life satisfaction and functioning rather than just reduced distress.

Quality of life assessment includes both objective measures (work performance, relationship stability, health behaviors) and subjective experiences (life satisfaction, meaning and purpose, emotional well-being). This comprehensive approach ensures that therapeutic gains translate into real-world improvements in daily living.

Case Example: Sarah's Holistic Progress Evaluation

Sarah, a 28-year-old teacher, completed quarterly quality of life assessments that revealed the broader impact of her schema work beyond specific symptom improvement. Her systematic evaluation showed how Abandonment and Emotional Deprivation schema healing affected multiple life areas.

Sarah's quality of life tracking included several domains:

186

Relationship Satisfaction: Sarah rated her satisfaction with friendships, family relationships, and romantic connections. Her scores showed steady improvement as she became more authentic in relationships and less fearful of abandonment, leading to deeper and more satisfying connections.

Work Fulfillment: Sarah measured job satisfaction, stress levels, and sense of professional competence. Her scores improved significantly as she stopped seeking excessive reassurance from supervisors and began trusting her own judgment about teaching decisions.

Physical Health: Sarah tracked sleep quality, exercise habits, nutrition choices, and medical care compliance. Her health behaviors improved as she reduced anxiety-related insomnia and stress eating while increasing self-care activities.

Emotional Well-being: Sarah assessed mood stability, anxiety levels, emotional regulation capacity, and overall psychological comfort. Her scores showed dramatic improvement in emotional stability and reduced anxiety.

Personal Growth: Sarah evaluated her sense of progress toward personal goals, learning and development activities, and feelings of self-efficacy. Her scores increased as she gained confidence in her ability to create positive changes.

Social Connection: Sarah measured the quality and quantity of her social relationships, community involvement, and sense of belonging. Her scores improved as she became more socially engaged and less isolated.

Life Meaning: Sarah assessed her sense of purpose, value alignment, and overall life satisfaction. Her scores showed steady improvement as she became more authentic and self-directed.

The comprehensive assessment revealed that Sarah's therapeutic gains were translating into broad life improvements rather than just specific symptom relief.

Assessment Implementation Approach

Include both subjective satisfaction ratings and objective behavioral indicators for each life domain: how satisfied you feel and what evidence supports those feelings.

Rate each domain on consistent scales (typically 1-10) that allow for comparison across time and identification of relative strengths and challenges.

Complete assessments quarterly or semi-annually to capture meaningful changes without creating assessment burden. More frequent assessment may show too much normal fluctuation.

Compare assessment results across time periods to identify improvement trends, persistent challenges, and life areas that may need additional attention.

Use assessment results to guide therapeutic priority setting and goal development: areas with consistently low scores may benefit from targeted intervention.

Exercise 74: Relationship Quality Tracker

Monitoring Interpersonal Improvements

The Relationship Quality Tracker focuses specifically on improvements in interpersonal relationships—often the most important outcome area for people working on relationship schemas. This tool measures both the quality of existing relationships and changes in your capacity to form new, healthy connections. Relationship tracking helps identify which therapeutic gains translate into improved interpersonal functioning.

Effective relationship tracking includes both your experience of relationships (satisfaction, trust, intimacy) and behavioral changes in how you interact with others (communication, boundary setting, conflict resolution). This dual focus ensures that internal changes translate into external relationship improvements.

Case Example: Michael's Social Connection Renaissance

Michael, a 35-year-old engineer, used relationship quality tracking to monitor his progress in addressing Social Isolation and Mistrust schemas that had left him with superficial connections and chronic loneliness. His systematic tracking revealed significant improvements in both relationship quality and quantity.

Michael's relationship tracking included several categories:

Friendship Quality: Michael rated the depth, satisfaction, and reliability of his friendships on a monthly basis. His scores showed steady improvement as he became more authentic and vulnerable with trusted friends, leading to deeper and more supportive connections.

Family Relationships: Michael assessed his relationships with family members, including communication frequency, emotional connection, and conflict resolution. His scores improved as he set healthier boundaries while increasing emotional availability.

Romantic Relationships: Michael tracked his dating experiences and romantic relationship satisfaction. His scores showed improvement in his ability to maintain authentic relationships without either excessive neediness or emotional withdrawal.

Professional Relationships: Michael measured workplace relationship satisfaction, collaboration effectiveness, and social comfort in professional settings. His scores improved as he became more socially engaged at work and less fearful of colleague interactions.

Social Activities: Michael tracked his participation in social events, group activities, and community involvement. His behavioral changes showed steady increases in social engagement and decreased isolation behaviors.

Communication Skills: Michael assessed his comfort with emotional expression, conflict resolution, and intimate conversation. His skills showed consistent improvement as he practiced vulnerability and authentic communication.

Trust and Intimacy: Michael measured his capacity for trusting others and allowing emotional closeness. His scores showed gradual but significant improvement in his ability to form close bonds without excessive fear or suspicion.

The tracking revealed that Michael's relationship improvements occurred gradually but consistently, with social skills gains preceding deeper intimacy improvements.

Relationship Tracking Framework

Focus on both relationship quality (satisfaction, trust, intimacy) and relationship quantity (frequency of contact, number of close relationships, social activity participation).

Include different types of relationships rather than focusing only on romantic partnerships: friendships, family relationships, professional connections, and community relationships all provide valuable information.

Track both your experience of relationships and others' responses to your interpersonal changes: how you feel about relationships and how others seem to experience you.

Monitor specific relationship skills that your schema work targets: communication, conflict resolution, boundary setting, emotional expression, and trust building.

Include behavioral indicators that reflect relationship improvements: frequency of social contact, depth of conversations, conflict resolution success, and support-seeking behavior.

Exercise 75: Therapist Progress Notes Template

Structured Documentation

The Therapist Progress Notes Template provides a systematic framework for mental health professionals to document client progress, track therapeutic interventions, and plan future treatment directions. Effective progress notes serve multiple functions: they provide legal documentation of services provided, track client progress over time, guide treatment planning decisions, and facilitate communication between providers when necessary.

Professional progress notes must balance comprehensiveness with efficiency, providing sufficient detail to support quality care while remaining practical to complete within typical session time constraints. The template ensures that essential information gets documented consistently while allowing for individualized observations and clinical insights.

Case Example: Dr. Martinez's Schema Therapy Documentation System

Dr. Martinez, a licensed clinical psychologist, developed a streamlined progress note template specifically designed for schema therapy work that efficiently captured essential therapeutic information while supporting treatment planning and outcome measurement.

Dr. Martinez's template included several key sections:

Session Overview: Brief description of session focus, primary interventions used, and client's general presentation and engagement level during the session.

Schema Work: Specific schemas addressed during the session, any new schema activation patterns identified, and client's current understanding and awareness of schema patterns.

Mode Work: Observations about client's mode functioning during session, any mode transitions observed, and progress in accessing

191

Healthy Adult mode during session or reported from between-session periods.

Therapeutic Interventions: Specific techniques used during session (imagery rescripting, chair work, cognitive restructuring), client's response to interventions, and effectiveness of different approaches.

Homework and Between-Session Work: Assignments given, client's compliance with previous homework, and any significant between-session experiences related to therapeutic goals.

Progress Indicators: Observable changes in client functioning, behavior, or schema patterns since previous session, and any setbacks or challenges that emerged.

Treatment Planning: Priorities for future sessions, any needed adjustments to treatment approach or goals, and plans for addressing obstacles or challenges that emerged.

The template allowed Dr. Martinez to document sessions efficiently while maintaining focus on schema-specific therapeutic elements and ensuring that progress tracking information was systematically captured.

Documentation Template Development

Include sections that capture the essential elements of schema therapy work: schema patterns, mode functioning, therapeutic interventions, and progress indicators specific to this treatment approach.

Balance detail with efficiency to ensure notes can be completed within reasonable time constraints without sacrificing important clinical information.

Incorporate progress measurement elements that support outcome evaluation and treatment planning: behavioral changes, symptom improvement, and functional gains.

Include space for clinical observations and insights that support case conceptualization and treatment planning beyond basic session documentation.

Ensure template meets legal and ethical documentation requirements while serving clinical purposes: sufficient detail for continuity of care and treatment justification.

Building Evidence for Healing

Progress tracking transforms the subjective experience of therapeutic change into objective evidence that supports continued growth and healing. The tools in this section provide systematic approaches to measuring improvement across multiple domains while maintaining motivation during challenging periods. Effective progress tracking creates positive feedback loops that reinforce therapeutic gains while identifying areas needing additional attention.

The measurement process itself often contributes to therapeutic progress by increasing awareness of subtle changes that might otherwise go unnoticed. Regular tracking helps clients recognize patterns in their healing process, identify effective interventions, and maintain perspective during inevitable setbacks and plateau periods.

Perhaps most importantly, progress tracking provides evidence that change is possible even when current experience feels static or discouraging. The accumulation of small improvements over time creates compelling proof that therapeutic work produces meaningful results, supporting continued investment in the healing process even during difficult periods.

The Power of Perspective

Consistent progress tracking often reveals that healing happens more quickly and completely than subjective experience suggests. Clients frequently underestimate their improvement because they adapt to new functioning levels quickly, making previous difficulties feel distant and minimized. Systematic measurement provides objective evidence that challenges these minimizing tendencies and supports accurate assessment of therapeutic gains.

The tracking process also helps identify which interventions produce the most benefit for individual clients, allowing for treatment customization and efficiency improvements. Some clients respond better to cognitive work while others benefit more from experiential interventions. Progress data helps guide these clinical decisions based on evidence rather than assumptions.

Core Principles for Measuring Change

- Weekly schema progress reviews provide regular assessment of changes across multiple domains affected by schema healing work
- Goal setting and achievement tracking transforms abstract healing concepts into specific, measurable objectives that create motivation and direction
- Therapy milestone celebrations reinforce positive changes through recognition while building motivation for continued growth efforts
- Setback recovery planning normalizes temporary obstacles while providing specific strategies for learning from and overcoming challenges
- Quality of life assessment measures broader therapeutic impact beyond symptom reduction to include life satisfaction and functioning improvements
- Relationship quality tracking focuses on interpersonal gains that often represent the most meaningful outcomes for relationship schema work
- Therapist progress notes provide professional documentation that supports treatment planning and outcome evaluation
- Systematic tracking creates objective evidence of change that challenges subjective minimizing tendencies and supports continued therapeutic investment

Chapter 12: Self-Help and Maintenance Resources

Therapeutic breakthroughs mean little if they can't be sustained in daily life. The transition from intensive therapy to independent functioning represents one of the most challenging aspects of schema healing work—maintaining progress while navigating life's inevitable stresses without the regular support and guidance of a therapeutic relationship. The exercises in this section provide tools for ongoing self-care, crisis management, and continued growth that support long-term recovery and resilience[56].

Self-help and maintenance work requires a different skill set than active therapy. Instead of exploring and processing schemas intensively, maintenance involves recognizing when schemas are becoming activated and responding quickly with appropriate interventions. Instead of major therapeutic breakthroughs, maintenance focuses on small, consistent actions that prevent regression and support continued growth over months and years.

The maintenance phase of schema work often determines whether therapeutic gains translate into lasting life changes or gradually fade back to old patterns. These tools provide structured approaches to maintaining progress while building the skills needed for lifelong emotional health and relationship satisfaction.

Exercise 76: Daily Schema Maintenance Routine

Ongoing Self-Care Practices

Daily Schema Maintenance Routines create consistent practices that support emotional regulation, prevent schema activation, and maintain therapeutic gains through regular self-care activities. These routines work by addressing schema triggers proactively rather than reactively, building resilience through consistent positive practices, and maintaining connection to therapeutic insights and skills through daily reinforcement.

Effective maintenance routines balance structure with flexibility, providing consistent support while adapting to changing life circumstances. The routine should feel sustainable and nourishing rather than burdensome or rigid, supporting long-term adherence through genuine benefit rather than forced compliance.

Case Example: Patricia's Morning and Evening Practice

Patricia, a 36-year-old social worker, developed a daily maintenance routine that addressed her Self-Sacrifice and Approval-Seeking schemas through consistent self-care and boundary-reinforcement practices. Her routine evolved over time to include elements that provided both immediate benefit and long-term schema prevention.

Patricia's morning routine included several schema-focused elements:

Intention Setting: Patricia spent five minutes each morning connecting with her values and priorities for the day, reminding herself that her needs and preferences matter and deserve consideration in daily decisions.

Boundary Affirmation: Patricia reviewed her boundaries and limits, reminding herself of her right to say no, ask for help, and prioritize her own wellbeing alongside caring for others.

Energy Assessment: Patricia honestly assessed her physical and emotional energy levels, using this information to make realistic decisions about what she could handle during the day without depleting herself.

Gratitude Practice: Patricia identified three things she appreciated about her life, including at least one acknowledgment of something she had done well or a boundary she had maintained.

Patricia's evening routine provided reflection and integration:

Schema Check-In: Patricia reviewed the day for any moments of schema activation, celebrating successful responses and learning from situations where she fell back into old patterns.

196

Boundary Review: Patricia assessed how well she had maintained her boundaries during the day, expressing appreciation for successful limit-setting and identifying adjustments needed for future situations.

Self-Compassion Practice: Patricia offered herself kindness for any mistakes or struggles during the day, treating herself with the same understanding she would offer a good friend.

Tomorrow's Intentions: Patricia identified one specific way she would prioritize her own needs or maintain boundaries the following day, creating concrete plans rather than vague intentions.

The routine took about 15 minutes total and provided consistent support for Patricia's schema work while maintaining flexibility for busy or unusual days.

Routine Development Framework

Choose routine elements that directly address your specific schema patterns rather than generic self-care activities. Personalized practices provide more targeted support and feel more meaningful.

Include both preventive elements (practices that reduce schema activation risk) and responsive elements (tools for handling activation when it occurs).

Start with brief routines that feel sustainable rather than ambitious practices that become burdensome. Success with smaller routines builds confidence for expansion over time.

Include flexibility for different life circumstances: travel routines, busy day modifications, and emergency versions that maintain core elements when time is limited.

Review and adjust routines periodically based on changing needs, life circumstances, and evolving understanding of your schema patterns.

Exercise 77: Schema Emergency Plan

Crisis Intervention Strategies

Schema Emergency Plans provide specific protocols for handling intense schema activation that threatens to overwhelm your coping capacity or trigger destructive behaviors. These plans work by providing predetermined responses to crisis situations, reducing the need for decision-making when emotional capacity is compromised, and ensuring that effective interventions are available when they're most needed.

Emergency plans differ from daily maintenance routines by focusing on crisis management rather than prevention. They provide immediate stabilization strategies, safety protocols, and step-by-step procedures for handling emotional emergencies that might otherwise lead to harmful behaviors or therapeutic setbacks.

Case Example: James's Abandonment Crisis Protocol

James, a 33-year-old engineer, developed a comprehensive emergency plan for managing severe Abandonment schema activation that had previously led to destructive behaviors like excessive calling, showing up uninvited at his girlfriend's workplace, and threatening self-harm to prevent perceived rejection.

James's emergency plan included several escalating levels of intervention:

Level 1 - Early Warning Response (when abandonment fears start but haven't overwhelmed coping capacity):

- Use grounding techniques to stay present rather than projecting into feared future scenarios
- Review evidence of relationship stability and partner's consistent caring behavior
- Call crisis support person for reality check and emotional support
- Engage in physical activity to discharge anxiety energy
- Set timer for 2 hours before taking any relationship-focused action

Level 2 - Moderate Crisis Response (when abandonment panic is strong but manageable):

- Implement complete contact moratorium with partner for 24 hours to prevent impulsive actions
- Use intensive self-soothing techniques including hot bath, comfort food, soothing music
- Write letter expressing all fears and feelings without sending it
- Practice radical acceptance that uncertainty is part of all relationships
- Contact therapist for emergency session if crisis doesn't resolve within 24 hours

Level 3 - Severe Crisis Response (when abandonment terror feels overwhelming and destructive urges emerge):

- Call crisis hotline immediately for professional support
- Remove means for impulsive contact with partner (give phone to trusted friend)
- Go to safe location with supportive person who understands the situation
- Use intensive grounding techniques and consider emergency medication if prescribed
- Implement safety plan to prevent self-harm or other destructive behaviors

James's plan also included contact information for crisis resources, written reminders of coping skills, and specific instructions for trusted friends about how to provide support during abandonment crises.

Emergency Plan Development

Identify your specific crisis triggers and early warning signs that indicate emergency intervention may be needed. Different schemas have different crisis patterns that require tailored responses.

Create escalating levels of intervention that match different crisis intensities rather than one-size-fits-all approaches that may be insufficient for severe episodes.

Include immediate safety measures that prevent harmful behaviors during emotional overwhelm: contact restrictions, means limitation, and professional support access.

Prepare emergency resources in advance when you're calm and thinking clearly: contact lists, coping skill reminders, and safety items that support crisis management.

Practice emergency plan elements during calm periods so they're familiar and accessible during actual crises when cognitive capacity may be compromised.

Exercise 78: Self-Therapy Session Structure

Independent Work Guidelines

Self-Therapy Session Structure provides a framework for conducting meaningful therapeutic work independently, allowing for continued growth and processing without ongoing professional therapy. These sessions help maintain therapeutic momentum, process new challenges as they arise, and deepen insights gained during formal therapy through continued self-reflection and skill practice.

Independent therapy sessions require more structure than informal self-reflection to ensure they're productive and safe. The framework provides clear procedures for self-assessment, goal setting, intervention implementation, and progress evaluation that mirror professional therapy processes.

Case Example: Michelle's Monthly Self-Therapy Practice

Michelle, a 29-year-old teacher, established monthly self-therapy sessions to maintain progress in her Perfectionism and Self-Sacrifice schema work after completing formal therapy. Her structured approach helped her continue growing while managing new challenges independently.

Michelle's self-therapy session structure included several consistent elements:

Opening Assessment (15 minutes): Michelle reviewed her current functioning across multiple life areas, identifying any recent schema activation patterns, new challenges or stressors, and areas where she felt stuck or needed additional work.

Goal Identification (10 minutes): Michelle selected 1-2 specific issues to focus on during the session, choosing problems that felt manageable for independent work rather than overwhelming challenges that might require professional support.

Intervention Implementation (30 minutes): Michelle used specific therapeutic techniques she'd learned during formal therapy, including chair work for internal conflicts, cognitive restructuring for problematic thinking patterns, and imagery work for emotional processing.

Skill Practice (15 minutes): Michelle practiced new behaviors or coping strategies, often through role-playing, writing exercises, or planning specific behavioral experiments for the coming month.

Integration and Planning (10 minutes): Michelle summarized insights gained during the session, identified specific actions to take based on the work, and planned follow-up activities to maintain momentum from the session.

Michelle's sessions provided ongoing therapeutic benefit while helping her maintain connection to her healing work and continue developing her emotional health skills independently.

Session Structure Development

Set consistent time limits for different session elements to ensure balanced attention to assessment, intervention, and integration rather than spending entire sessions on single activities.

Choose intervention techniques that are safe and appropriate for independent use rather than attempting complex or potentially destabilizing therapeutic work without professional support.

Include both problem-focused work (addressing current challenges) and growth-focused activities (building new skills and expanding capacity) for balanced development.

Document session insights and plans to track patterns over time and ensure follow-through on therapeutic work between sessions.

Establish clear criteria for when self-therapy sessions aren't sufficient and professional support should be sought for additional challenges or complex issues.

Exercise 79: Schema Affirmations and Mantras

Positive Self-Talk Development

Schema Affirmations and Mantras provide specific language for countering schema-driven negative self-talk with realistic, positive statements that support healthy self-concept and emotional regulation. These tools work by replacing automatic negative thoughts with deliberately chosen positive messages that reinforce therapeutic gains and support continued growth.

Effective affirmations differ from generic positive thinking by specifically addressing schema patterns and being grounded in realistic self-assessment rather than wishful thinking. They acknowledge current reality while supporting movement toward healthier patterns and self-concept.

Case Example: Robert's Truth-Based Affirmation System

Robert, a 41-year-old consultant, developed a system of schema-specific affirmations that addressed his Defectiveness and Failure schemas with realistic, evidence-based positive statements. His affirmations evolved from therapeutic insights and were grounded in actual experiences and achievements.

Robert's affirmation categories addressed different schema themes:

Worth and Lovability Affirmations (addressing Defectiveness schema):

- "I am worthy of love and respect exactly as I am, with both strengths and areas for growth"
- "My value as a person doesn't depend on my performance or achievements"
- "I have qualities that others appreciate and find valuable in relationships"
- "I deserve kindness and understanding, especially from myself"

Competence and Success Affirmations (addressing Failure schema):

- "I have successfully handled many challenges and learned from difficult experiences"
- "I have skills and knowledge that contribute value in my work and relationships"
- "Mistakes are opportunities for learning rather than evidence of incompetence"
- "I can handle uncertainty and challenges with resilience and creativity"

Growth and Change Affirmations (supporting ongoing healing):

- "I am capable of continued growth and positive change throughout my life"
- "I can learn new skills and develop healthier patterns of thinking and behaving"
- "My past experiences inform but don't limit my future possibilities"
- "I have the strength and wisdom to create the life I want"

Robert used these affirmations during morning routines, stressful situations, and times when schema-driven negative self-talk emerged. The evidence-based nature of the statements made them feel genuine and believable rather than forced or artificial.

Affirmation Development Process

Ground affirmations in actual evidence and experience rather than wishful thinking or generic positive statements. Believable affirmations have more impact than unrealistic declarations.

Address your specific schema patterns and negative self-talk themes rather than using general affirmations that may not target your particular challenges.

Include both current reality acknowledgments and growth-oriented statements that support movement toward healthier self-concept and functioning.

Create affirmations that feel authentic in your natural language and speaking style rather than formal or artificial phrasing that doesn't resonate emotionally.

Practice affirmations regularly during calm periods to strengthen their availability during schema activation when negative self-talk tends to emerge.

Exercise 80: Booster Session Activities

Periodic Check-In Exercises

Booster Session Activities provide structured opportunities for periodic intensive self-assessment and therapeutic work that support long-term maintenance and continued growth. These sessions work by identifying emerging challenges before they become overwhelming, reinforcing therapeutic gains through regular practice, and providing opportunities for deeper self-reflection that daily maintenance routines might not accommodate.

Booster sessions differ from regular self-therapy sessions by being more comprehensive and intensive, focusing on overall progress assessment and major life adjustments rather than specific current problems. They serve as periodic tune-ups that maintain therapeutic momentum and prevent gradual drift back toward old patterns.

Case Example: Lisa's Quarterly Growth Reviews

Lisa, a 32-year-old graphic designer, established quarterly booster sessions that provided comprehensive review of her schema healing progress and planning for continued growth. Her systematic approach helped maintain therapeutic gains while adapting to changing life circumstances.

Lisa's quarterly booster sessions included several comprehensive elements:

Progress Assessment (45 minutes): Lisa systematically reviewed her functioning across all life areas affected by her schema work, comparing current functioning to previous quarters and identifying areas of improvement and ongoing challenges.

Schema Pattern Review (30 minutes): Lisa examined her schema activation patterns over the previous three months, identifying triggers that continued to create difficulties and celebrating situations where she responded with healthy patterns.

Goal Evaluation and Setting (30 minutes): Lisa assessed progress on previous quarter's goals and established new objectives for the upcoming three months based on current needs and growth opportunities.

Skill Refresher (45 minutes): Lisa practiced therapeutic techniques she hadn't used recently, reviewed coping strategies that had been most helpful, and learned new skills that addressed emerging challenges.

Life Planning Integration (30 minutes): Lisa considered how her continued schema healing work fit with broader life goals and plans, ensuring that therapeutic insights informed major life decisions and directions.

Lisa's booster sessions provided intensive therapeutic work that maintained her healing momentum while helping her adapt her schema work to changing life circumstances and continued growth needs.

Booster Session Planning

Schedule booster sessions at regular intervals (quarterly or semi-annually) rather than waiting for crises or major problems to emerge. Preventive approach maintains momentum more effectively.

Include comprehensive assessment of multiple life areas rather than focusing only on problem areas. Balanced review provides perspective on overall progress and areas needing attention.

Combine review of past progress with planning for future growth to maintain both appreciation for achievements and motivation for continued development.

Include skill practice and learning elements that prevent therapeutic tools from becoming rusty through disuse and add new capabilities as understanding deepens.

Integrate schema work with broader life planning to ensure that healing insights inform major life decisions and directions rather than remaining separate from practical life management.

Exercise 81: Schema Recovery Milestones

Celebrating Long-Term Progress

Schema Recovery Milestones provide a framework for recognizing and celebrating significant achievements in long-term healing work that might otherwise go unnoticed in the focus on daily challenges and ongoing growth. These milestones work by creating specific markers of progress that can be celebrated and referenced during difficult periods, building identity as someone who has successfully changed difficult patterns, and providing motivation for continued growth through recognition of substantial achievements.

Recovery milestones differ from therapy milestones by focusing on long-term pattern changes and life improvements rather than short-term therapeutic gains. They recognize fundamental shifts in how you think, feel, and behave that represent genuine healing rather than temporary improvement.

Case Example: Sarah's Five-Year Transformation Recognition

Sarah, now 33 years old, celebrated the five-year anniversary of beginning intensive schema therapy work for her Abandonment and Emotional Deprivation schemas. Her milestone celebration recognized fundamental life changes that went far beyond symptom improvement to include genuine life transformation.

Sarah's milestone recognition included several reflection categories:

Relationship Transformation: Sarah compared her current relationship capacity to her functioning five years earlier. She had moved from isolated, superficial connections to a close marriage, several deep friendships, and improved family relationships. Her relationships were characterized by mutual support rather than anxiety-driven people-pleasing.

Emotional Regulation Growth: Sarah's emotional life had changed from chronic anxiety and depression with frequent emotional crises to stable mood with normal emotional fluctuations. She could handle relationship conflicts without panic and express needs without terror of abandonment.

Professional Development: Sarah's career had advanced from a job she tolerated to work she found meaningful and engaging. She had developed leadership skills and could handle workplace challenges without schema activation.

Self-Concept Evolution: Sarah's identity had shifted from seeing herself as fundamentally flawed and unlovable to understanding herself as someone with normal human strengths and challenges worthy of love and respect.

Life Satisfaction Improvement: Sarah's overall life satisfaction had increased dramatically, with genuine happiness and contentment replacing chronic anxiety and emptiness. She could envision positive futures and work toward meaningful goals.

Sarah's celebration included writing letters to her past self, sharing appreciation with people who had supported her healing, and committing to continued growth while honoring how far she had come.

Milestone Recognition Framework

Choose meaningful time intervals for milestone celebration (annual, five-year) that allow sufficient time for substantial changes to occur rather than minor improvements.

Include both internal changes (emotional regulation, self-concept, coping capacity) and external changes (relationships, career, life satisfaction) that demonstrate comprehensive healing.

Document specific examples and evidence of change rather than general impressions to create concrete recognition of actual transformation.

Share milestone celebrations with supportive people who can appreciate the significance of your growth and provide external validation of changes they've observed.

Use milestone recognition to inform future goals and directions while celebrating current achievements rather than immediately focusing on remaining challenges.

Exercise 82: Creating Your Personal Schema Toolkit

Customized Resource Collection

Creating Your Personal Schema Toolkit involves developing a comprehensive, personalized collection of resources, tools, and strategies that support your ongoing schema healing work. This toolkit serves as a portable therapeutic resource that can be accessed whenever challenges arise, providing immediate support for emotional regulation, crisis management, and continued growth.

The personal toolkit differs from generic self-help resources by being specifically tailored to your unique schema patterns, life circumstances, and therapeutic needs. It includes tools that have proven effective through personal experience rather than theoretical recommendations that may not match your individual healing process.

Case Example: Michael's Comprehensive Healing Arsenal

Michael, a 38-year-old marketing director, spent several months developing a comprehensive personal toolkit that addressed his Mistrust and Social Isolation schemas while supporting his continued growth and emotional health. His toolkit evolved over time as he discovered which resources provided the most benefit.

Michael's toolkit included several categories of resources:

Immediate Crisis Support: Contact list of crisis resources and supportive people, emergency coping skill reminders written on index cards, guided meditations on his phone for anxiety management, and specific instructions for handling severe mistrust episodes.

Daily Maintenance Tools: Morning and evening routine guidelines, boundary-setting language for common situations, self-compassion exercises for difficult days, and relationship skills reminders for social interactions.

Growth and Development Resources: Books and articles about trust-building and social connection, inspirational quotes and stories that reinforced healing goals, creative exercises for emotional expression, and learning opportunities for continued personal development.

Assessment and Tracking Materials: Weekly check-in forms for monitoring progress, goal-setting worksheets for planning continued growth, relationship satisfaction assessments for tracking interpersonal improvements, and journal prompts for ongoing self-reflection.

Environmental Supports: Photos and reminders of supportive relationships and positive experiences, comfortable items for self-soothing during difficult periods, organized living space that supported emotional regulation, and access to nature and beauty for mood enhancement.

Michael's toolkit provided comprehensive support for his ongoing healing work while remaining practical and accessible during daily life challenges and stressful periods.

Toolkit Development Process

Include resources for different types of challenges rather than focusing only on crisis management: daily maintenance, growth promotion, and specific skill development tools.

Choose tools that have proven effective through personal experience rather than collecting resources that seem theoretically helpful but haven't been tested in your life.

Organize toolkit elements for easy access during different types of situations: immediate crisis needs, ongoing support requirements, and growth-focused activities.

Include both independent resources (tools you can use alone) and social resources (people and activities that provide support and connection).

Review and update toolkit contents regularly as your needs change and you discover new resources that provide benefit for your continued healing work.

Building a Life Worth Living

The transition from therapeutic healing to independent living represents both an achievement and an ongoing responsibility. The tools in this section provide frameworks for maintaining therapeutic gains while continuing to grow and develop throughout your life. Schema healing isn't a destination but a foundation for continued personal development and life satisfaction.

The maintenance phase often determines whether therapeutic insights translate into lasting life changes or gradually fade back to familiar patterns. These resources provide structured approaches to ongoing self-care that prevent regression while supporting continued growth and adaptation to life's inevitable changes and challenges.

Perhaps most importantly, these tools help you develop the internal resources needed for lifelong emotional health rather than depending on external support for ongoing wellbeing. While supportive relationships and professional help remain valuable throughout life, the capacity for self-care and continued growth provides the foundation for sustained happiness and resilience.

The Journey Continues

Schema healing work represents the beginning rather than the end of a journey toward emotional health and life satisfaction. The patterns addressed through therapeutic work often took years or decades to develop, and their healing creates space for continued growth and development that extends far beyond symptom relief or problem resolution.

The self-help and maintenance resources in this section provide tools for navigating this ongoing journey with wisdom, compassion, and realistic expectations. They support the development of internal resources that can sustain you through life's inevitable challenges while creating opportunities for continued growth and positive change throughout your lifetime.

Essential Elements for Lifelong Wellbeing

- Daily schema maintenance routines provide consistent self-care practices that prevent schema activation while supporting ongoing emotional health
- Schema emergency plans ensure that crisis intervention strategies are available when emotional overwhelm threatens therapeutic progress
- Self-therapy session structures allow for continued growth and processing without ongoing professional therapy support
- Schema affirmations and mantras provide positive self-talk tools that counter negative thought patterns with realistic, evidence-based statements
- Booster session activities offer periodic intensive check-ins that maintain therapeutic momentum and adapt healing work to changing life circumstances
- Schema recovery milestones recognize and celebrate long-term achievements that might otherwise go unnoticed in daily life focus
- Personal schema toolkits provide comprehensive, customized resources for ongoing support that address individual needs and proven effective strategies
- Maintenance work transforms therapeutic insights into sustainable life practices that support continued growth and resilience throughout life

Chapter 13: Advanced Schema Therapy Techniques

Advanced Schema Therapy techniques require sophisticated understanding of schema dynamics and refined clinical skills to implement safely and effectively. These interventions go beyond basic cognitive, behavioral, and experiential work to address complex presentations, treatment-resistant patterns, and specialized populations[89]. Advanced techniques often combine multiple therapeutic elements while requiring careful attention to timing, client readiness, and potential for destabilization.

The development of advanced skills in Schema Therapy happens gradually through supervised practice, personal therapy experience, and ongoing professional development. These techniques aren't simply more complex versions of basic interventions—they represent qualitatively different approaches that address deeper levels of psychological organization and change.

Exercise 83: Multi-Modal Schema Integration

Combining Cognitive, Emotional, and Somatic Approaches Simultaneously

Multi-Modal Schema Integration involves using cognitive, emotional, and somatic interventions simultaneously to create powerful healing experiences that address schemas at multiple levels of psychological organization. This technique recognizes that schemas exist in thoughts, feelings, body sensations, and behavioral patterns that must be addressed together for lasting change.

Case Example: Elena's Trauma Integration Work

Elena, a 38-year-old therapist, used multi-modal integration to address her Vulnerability to Harm schema that developed from childhood sexual abuse. The work combined cognitive restructuring of safety beliefs with emotional processing of fear responses and somatic work to address body-based trauma reactions.

During one session, Elena worked cognitively to challenge catastrophic thoughts about current safety while simultaneously using breathing techniques to regulate her nervous system and chair work to dialogue between her frightened child part and protective adult self. The multi-modal approach addressed her schema at all levels of experience.

Implementation Framework:

- Identify which modalities most strongly maintain the target schema
- Design interventions that address cognitive, emotional, and somatic elements simultaneously
- Monitor for overwhelm while maximizing therapeutic impact
- Integrate insights across all modalities for complete understanding

Exercise 84: Schema Timeline Reconstruction

Mapping Schema Development Through Life Stages

Schema Timeline Reconstruction creates detailed maps of how specific schemas developed and changed throughout different life stages. This technique helps clients understand the adaptive logic of their schemas while identifying key developmental periods that require healing attention.

Case Example: Marcus's Abandonment Timeline

Marcus, a 45-year-old businessman, created a detailed timeline showing how his Abandonment schema developed from infancy through adulthood. The timeline revealed critical periods: father's departure at age 3, mother's emotional unavailability during depression, boarding school placement at age 12, and repeated relationship losses in early adulthood.

The timeline work helped Marcus understand that his schema wasn't irrational but represented logical adaptations to repeated experiences of loss and abandonment. Each life stage had reinforced the pattern while teaching him specific coping strategies that now required updating.

Exercise 85: Intergenerational Schema Mapping

Exploring Family Patterns Across Multiple Generations

Intergenerational Schema Mapping examines how schemas pass from one generation to the next through family patterns, cultural transmission, and learned coping strategies. This technique helps clients understand their schemas within broader family and cultural contexts while breaking cycles of intergenerational trauma.

Case Example: Sofia's Three-Generation Perfectionism Pattern

Sofia, a 32-year-old architect, mapped perfectionist patterns across three generations of her family. Her grandmother survived war and poverty through meticulous planning and flawless execution. Her mother inherited these patterns and added academic achievement pressure. Sofia carried both elements while adding professional performance anxiety.

The mapping helped Sofia appreciate the survival value of perfectionism in her family history while recognizing how circumstances had changed. She could honor her family's resilience while choosing more balanced approaches for her current life situation.

Exercise 86: Schema Dialogue with Multiple Parts

Complex Internal Conversations Between Various Schema Aspects

Schema Dialogue with Multiple Parts extends basic chair work to include conversations between multiple schema modes, healthy parts, and protective mechanisms simultaneously. This technique addresses complex internal systems where multiple schemas interact in sophisticated ways.

Case Example: David's Internal Family Meeting

David, a 39-year-old teacher, facilitated a dialogue between his Vulnerable Child (who felt inadequate), Demanding Parent (who pushed for perfection), Angry Child (who resented the pressure), and Healthy Adult (who sought balance). The multi-part dialogue revealed how these different aspects had been fighting against each other rather than working together.

The complex dialogue helped David's internal parts negotiate better relationships and establish his Healthy Adult as a wise coordinator rather than letting the Demanding Parent dominate all decisions.

Exercise 87: Corrective Relational Experiences

Structured Experiences That Contradict Schema Predictions

Corrective Relational Experiences involve carefully designed interpersonal interactions that directly contradict schema-based expectations about relationships. These experiences provide evidence that schemas may not be accurate in current circumstances while building new templates for healthy relationships.

Case Example: Jennifer's Trust Building Experiment

Jennifer, with severe Mistrust schemas from childhood abuse, engaged in a structured trust-building exercise with her therapy group. She shared increasingly personal information over several months while other members consistently responded with support rather than judgment or exploitation.

The corrective experience provided evidence that contradicted her schema's predictions about inevitable betrayal and harm from others.

Each positive interaction weakened her Mistrust schema while building new neural pathways for healthy relationships.

Exercise 88: Schema-Focused EMDR Integration

Combining Eye Movement Processing with Schema Work

Schema-Focused EMDR Integration combines EMDR's bilateral stimulation with schema-specific targets and positive cognitions. This approach addresses traumatic memories that formed schemas while installing healthier beliefs and emotional responses.

Case Example: Robert's Combat Trauma Schema Work

Robert, a 41-year-old veteran, used EMDR to process combat memories while targeting Vulnerability and Mistrust schemas that developed from war experiences. The bilateral stimulation helped process specific traumatic incidents while installing positive cognitions about current safety and trustworthiness of civilians.

The integration was more effective than either EMDR or Schema Therapy alone because it addressed both specific memories and general life patterns created by military trauma.

Exercise 89: Advanced Imagery Rescripting with Future Self

Meeting and Learning from Your Healed Future Self

Advanced Imagery Rescripting involves connecting with a future version of yourself who has successfully healed from current schema patterns. This technique provides hope, guidance, and concrete examples of healthy functioning while building motivation for continued healing work.

Case Example: Lisa's Future Self Guidance

Lisa, struggling with Self-Sacrifice schemas, met her future self at age 55 who had learned to balance caring for others with self-care. Her future self provided specific guidance about boundary setting, self-compassion, and maintaining relationships while honoring personal needs.

The imagery work inspired Lisa while providing concrete examples of how her life could be different. Her future self became an internal resource she could access during difficult decisions about self-care and boundaries.

Exercise 90: Schema Constellation Work

Using Spatial Positioning to Explore Schema Relationships

Schema Constellation Work uses physical positioning in space to explore relationships between different schemas, family members, and internal parts. This technique makes abstract psychological relationships concrete and visible while revealing hidden dynamics and connections.

Case Example: Michael's Family Schema Constellation

Michael arranged chairs representing family members and his various schemas in physical space, then moved between positions to understand their relationships. He discovered that his Emotional Deprivation schema stood between him and other family members, protecting him from further disappointment while preventing connection.

The constellation work revealed spatial and emotional dynamics that weren't obvious through talking alone, providing new understanding of how his schemas functioned as protective barriers.

Chapter 14: Specialized Populations and Adaptations

Schema Therapy principles remain consistent across populations, but their application requires careful adaptation to different developmental stages, cultural contexts, and specific needs. Working with specialized populations demands understanding of how schemas manifest differently in various groups while maintaining fidelity to core therapeutic principles[90].

Each population brings unique considerations regarding assessment methods, intervention techniques, therapeutic relationships, and treatment goals. Successful adaptation requires deep understanding of both Schema Therapy principles and the specific characteristics and needs of different populations.

Exercise 91: Adolescent Schema Assessment

Age-Appropriate Evaluation for Developing Personalities

Adolescent Schema Assessment adapts standard schema evaluation for developing personalities where schemas are still forming and more fluid than in adults. This assessment considers normal developmental processes while identifying problematic patterns that require intervention.

Case Example: Tyler's Emerging Perfectionism

Tyler, a 16-year-old high school student, showed signs of developing Unrelenting Standards schema through academic pressure and social comparison. The assessment revealed that his perfectionism was intensifying during the stress of college preparation and social media exposure to others' achievements.

The adolescent-adapted assessment considered Tyler's developmental stage while identifying concerning patterns that could benefit from early intervention before becoming entrenched adult schemas.

Adaptation Guidelines:

- Consider normal adolescent development versus problematic patterns
- Involve family members while respecting adolescent autonomy
- Use age-appropriate language and examples
- Focus on prevention and early intervention rather than established patterns

Exercise 92: Couples Schema Interaction Mapping

Understanding How Partner Schemas Trigger Each Other

Couples Schema Interaction Mapping examines how each partner's schemas trigger and reinforce the other's patterns, creating negative cycles that damage relationships. This technique helps couples understand their interactions at schema levels rather than surface behavioral conflicts.

Case Example: Sarah and Mike's Pursuer-Distancer Cycle

Sarah's Abandonment schema made her pursue connection when Mike seemed distant, while Mike's Emotional Deprivation schema made him withdraw when Sarah seemed demanding. Their schemas created a cycle where each partner's behavior confirmed the other's worst fears.

The mapping helped both partners understand that their conflicts reflected schema triggers rather than personal attacks, allowing them to respond to each other's underlying needs rather than defensive behaviors.

Mapping Process:

- Identify each partner's primary schemas
- Map how these schemas interact during conflicts
- Understand the protective function of each partner's responses

- Develop alternatives that meet both partners' schema needs

Exercise 93: Cultural Schema Adaptation

Modifying Techniques for Different Cultural Contexts

Cultural Schema Adaptation involves modifying Schema Therapy techniques to be appropriate and effective across different cultural contexts. This includes understanding how schemas manifest differently in various cultures while adapting interventions to cultural values and practices.

Case Example: Amara's Collectivist Family Values

Amara, from a collectivist culture, struggled with what appeared to be Self-Sacrifice schema but was actually healthy cultural expression of family responsibility. The cultural adaptation helped distinguish between problematic self-sacrifice and appropriate cultural values.

The adapted approach honored Amara's cultural values while addressing the specific aspects of her self-sacrifice that created personal distress and relationship problems within her cultural context.

Cultural Considerations:

- Understand how schemas manifest differently across cultures
- Adapt assessment tools for cultural appropriateness
- Modify interventions to align with cultural values
- Include cultural strengths and resources in treatment

Exercise 94: Schema Work with Trauma Survivors

Specialized Approaches for Complex Trauma Presentations

Schema Work with Trauma Survivors requires careful attention to safety, pacing, and stabilization while addressing the complex schema

221

patterns that often develop from traumatic experiences. This approach integrates trauma-informed care with schema healing.

Case Example: Maria's Complex Trauma Recovery

Maria, a survivor of childhood abuse, developed multiple schemas including Mistrust, Vulnerability to Harm, and Defectiveness. The trauma-informed approach focused on safety and stabilization before addressing schema patterns, using grounding techniques and careful pacing throughout treatment.

The specialized approach helped Maria heal from both specific traumatic experiences and the broader life patterns that trauma had created, addressing both past wounds and current functioning.

Trauma-Informed Adaptations:

- Prioritize safety and stabilization before schema processing
- Use grounding techniques throughout therapy sessions
- Address dissociation and emotional regulation before deeper work
- Coordinate with trauma specialists and other providers as needed

Exercise 95: Group Schema Psychoeducation

Teaching Schema Concepts to Multiple Participants

Group Schema Psychoeducation provides structured learning experiences that help multiple participants understand schema concepts while building group cohesion and mutual support. This approach uses group dynamics to enhance individual learning and healing.

Case Example: The Anxiety Support Group's Schema Education

A group of eight people with anxiety disorders learned about Vulnerability to Harm and Unrelenting Standards schemas through interactive exercises, shared examples, and mutual support. The group format helped normalize schema experiences while providing multiple perspectives on healing.

The psychoeducation approach helped group members understand their anxiety through schema frameworks while building supportive relationships with others who shared similar patterns.

Group Education Elements:

- Present schema concepts in accessible, interactive formats
- Encourage sharing and mutual support around schema experiences
- Use group dynamics to normalize and validate schema patterns
- Provide homework and practice opportunities between sessions

Exercise 96: Schema Therapy for Eating Disorders

Addressing Body Image and Food Schemas

Schema Therapy for Eating Disorders addresses the underlying schema patterns that often maintain disordered eating behaviors. This approach goes beyond symptom management to address core beliefs about self-worth, control, and body image.

Case Example: Jessica's Perfectionism and Body Image

Jessica's eating disorder was maintained by Unrelenting Standards and Defectiveness schemas that created impossible body image standards and self-worth based on appearance and control. Schema work addressed these underlying patterns while coordinating with nutritional and medical treatment.

The schema approach helped Jessica understand how her eating disorder served schema functions while developing healthier ways to meet her needs for control, self-worth, and emotional regulation.

Eating Disorder Adaptations:

- Address underlying schema patterns maintaining eating behaviors
- Coordinate with nutritional rehabilitation and medical care
- Focus on body image schemas and perfectionist patterns
- Integrate family work when appropriate for recovery support

Chapter 15: Research and Evidence Base

Schema Therapy's research foundation continues growing through controlled trials, effectiveness studies, and outcome research across diverse populations and settings. Understanding this evidence base helps practitioners stay current with research developments while maintaining evidence-based practice standards[91].

The research demonstrates Schema Therapy's effectiveness for personality disorders, treatment-resistant conditions, and complex presentations that may not respond adequately to other therapeutic approaches. This evidence supports Schema Therapy's position as an established, evidence-based treatment for difficult-to-treat conditions.

Exercise 97: Outcome Measurement in Schema Therapy

Systematic Evaluation of Treatment Effectiveness

Outcome Measurement involves systematic evaluation of Schema Therapy effectiveness using standardized instruments and regular assessment. This approach ensures accountability while providing feedback for treatment planning and modification.

Case Example: Dr. Peterson's Practice-Based Evidence

Dr. Peterson implemented systematic outcome measurement in her Schema Therapy practice, using pre-treatment, mid-treatment, and post-treatment assessments with standardized instruments. The data showed significant improvements in schema patterns, symptom reduction, and life satisfaction across her client population.

The measurement system helped Dr. Peterson identify which interventions were most effective for different client presentations while providing evidence of treatment effectiveness for insurance and accountability purposes.

Measurement Components:

- Pre-treatment assessment of schema patterns and functioning
- Regular progress monitoring throughout treatment
- Post-treatment evaluation of outcomes and maintenance
- Long-term follow-up to assess sustained improvement

Exercise 98: Schema Therapy Research Participation

Contributing to Evidence Base Through Clinical Research

Research Participation involves contributing to Schema Therapy's evidence base through participation in clinical trials, effectiveness studies, or practice-based research. This contribution advances the field while often providing enhanced treatment for research participants.

Case Example: Community Clinic Research Partnership

A community mental health clinic partnered with a university research center to study Schema Therapy effectiveness for clients with personality disorders. The research provided additional supervision and resources while contributing to evidence about Schema Therapy in community settings.

The partnership benefited both clients (who received enhanced treatment) and the field (which gained evidence about real-world effectiveness).

Research Considerations:

- Understand ethical requirements for research participation
- Ensure research enhances rather than compromises clinical care
- Contribute to evidence base while maintaining client welfare
- Use research findings to improve clinical practice

Exercise 99: Evidence-Based Practice Integration

Incorporating Research Findings into Clinical Work

226

Evidence-Based Practice Integration involves systematically incorporating research findings into Schema Therapy practice while maintaining attention to individual client needs and preferences. This approach balances research evidence with clinical expertise and client values.

Case Example: Implementing Research-Supported Modifications

Dr. Martinez modified her Schema Therapy approach based on research showing enhanced effectiveness when mindfulness techniques were integrated with traditional schema interventions. She systematically implemented these modifications while monitoring client responses and outcomes.

The integration improved treatment effectiveness while maintaining fidelity to evidence-based practice principles.

Integration Guidelines:

- Stay current with Schema Therapy research developments
- Implement research-supported modifications systematically
- Monitor client responses to evidence-based changes
- Balance research findings with individual client needs

Schema Therapy continues evolving through technological innovations, theoretical developments, and expanded applications. Understanding emerging trends helps practitioners prepare for future developments while contributing to the field's continued growth[92].

Future directions include technology integration, cultural adaptations, prevention applications, and expanded theoretical frameworks that build upon Schema Therapy's foundation while addressing new challenges and opportunities.

Exercise 100: Technology-Enhanced Schema Therapy

Integrating Digital Tools with Traditional Interventions

Technology-Enhanced Schema Therapy involves thoughtful integration of digital tools, apps, and platforms with traditional therapeutic interventions. This approach maintains the relational foundation of Schema Therapy while using technology to enhance accessibility, engagement, and effectiveness.

Case Example: Virtual Reality Exposure for Schemas

Dr. Thompson integrated virtual reality technology with Schema Therapy to help clients with Social Isolation schemas practice social interactions in safe, controlled environments. The VR exposure helped clients build confidence before applying skills in real-world situations.

The technology enhanced traditional Schema Therapy by providing additional practice opportunities while maintaining focus on therapeutic relationship and emotional processing.

Technology Integration Principles:

- Use technology to enhance rather than replace therapeutic relationships
- Maintain privacy and security in digital therapeutic tools
- Integrate technology thoughtfully with traditional interventions
- Monitor effectiveness of technology-enhanced approaches

Appendix A: 20 Early Maladaptive Schemas with Definitions

Schema identification requires precise understanding of each pattern's unique characteristics and manifestations. The 20 Early Maladaptive Schemas represent the most common dysfunctional patterns that develop when core childhood needs go unmet[83]. These schemas organize into five domains based on the fundamental needs they represent, creating a systematic framework for understanding how early experiences shape adult psychological functioning.

Each schema includes specific beliefs about yourself, others, and the world that create predictable emotional and behavioral patterns. Understanding these definitions helps you recognize your own schema patterns while appreciating how different combinations create unique individual presentations. The revised list includes two additional schemas identified through recent research, bringing the total from 18 to 20 patterns.

Domain I: Disconnection and Rejection

This domain includes schemas that develop when needs for safety, stability, love, and acceptance go unmet. People with these schemas expect that their needs for connection and emotional support will not be met in predictable or stable ways.

1. Abandonment/Instability Schema The belief that significant others will not continue providing emotional support and connection because they are emotionally unstable, unreliable, or unpredictable. This schema includes fears that loved ones will die, leave for someone better, or abandon you because you're somehow inadequate.

People with this schema often feel anxious in relationships, constantly scanning for signs of withdrawal or rejection. They may become clingy and demanding, ironically pushing people away through the very behaviors designed to prevent abandonment. The schema creates hypersensitivity to any changes in others' availability or mood.

Case Example: Maria becomes panicked when her boyfriend doesn't respond to texts within an hour, interpreting delays as evidence that he's losing interest. She feels compelled to call repeatedly or drive by his workplace to confirm he still cares, despite his consistent reassurance over their two-year relationship.

2. Mistrust/Abuse Schema The expectation that others will hurt, abuse, humiliate, cheat, manipulate, or take advantage of you. This schema involves constant vigilance for signs of mistreatment and difficulty trusting others' motivations, even in benign situations.

This pattern often develops from experiences of actual abuse or betrayal, creating a worldview where other people are fundamentally dangerous or exploitative. The schema makes it difficult to form close relationships due to constant suspicion and defensive positioning.

Case Example: David scrutinizes every interaction with colleagues for hidden agendas, interpreting friendly gestures as manipulation attempts. He avoids sharing personal information and keeps detailed mental records of others' behavior to protect himself from perceived threats that rarely materialize.

3. Emotional Deprivation Schema The belief that your emotional needs will never be adequately met by others. This includes deprivation of nurturance (lack of attention and affection), empathy (lack of understanding and listening), and protection (lack of guidance and direction from others).

People with this schema often feel emotionally hungry and empty, but may not express their needs directly due to beliefs that others can't or won't meet them. They may become withdrawn or overly self-reliant to avoid disappointment.

Case Example: Jennifer never asks friends for emotional support during difficult times, believing that others are too busy or don't really care about her problems. She maintains superficial relationships while feeling chronically lonely and misunderstood.

4. Defectiveness/Shame Schema The belief that you are defective, bad, unwanted, or inferior in important ways. This schema involves feeling flawed at your core and believing that if others knew the "real" you, they would reject you completely.

This pattern creates chronic shame and self-criticism, along with fears of exposure and rejection. People with this schema often hide their true selves and may be perfectionistic to compensate for perceived inadequacies.

Case Example: Robert believes something is fundamentally wrong with him and carefully manages his image to prevent others from discovering his "true" inadequate self. He avoids intimate relationships and social situations where his perceived flaws might be exposed.

5. Social Isolation/Alienation Schema The feeling that you are isolated from the world, different from other people, and don't belong to any group or community. This schema involves feeling like an outsider who can't fit in or connect with others.

People with this schema often feel lonely even in groups and may avoid social situations due to feeling fundamentally different or disconnected from others. They may prefer solitary activities and struggle with feelings of not belonging anywhere.

Case Example: Lisa feels like an alien observing human behavior from the outside, unable to understand social nuances or feel genuine connection with groups. She attends social events but feels invisible and disconnected, leading to increased isolation and withdrawal.

Domain II: Impaired Autonomy and Performance

This domain includes schemas that interfere with your ability to function independently and perform successfully. These patterns often develop in families that are overprotective, enmeshed, or that undermine confidence and independence.

6. Dependence/Incompetence Schema The belief that you cannot handle everyday responsibilities competently without considerable help from others. This schema involves feeling incompetent and needing others to help with decisions and daily functioning.

People with this schema often avoid challenges and may seek excessive advice and reassurance from others. They may feel overwhelmed by normal adult responsibilities and doubt their ability to manage independently.

Case Example: Michael seeks his mother's approval for all major decisions despite being 35 years old. He feels paralyzed when facing new challenges and immediately calls family members for guidance rather than trusting his own judgment.

7. Vulnerability to Harm or Illness Schema The exaggerated fear that catastrophe will strike at any time and that you cannot protect yourself. This includes fears of natural disasters, crime, accidents, or serious illness affecting yourself or loved ones.

This schema creates chronic anxiety and hypervigilance about potential dangers. People may engage in excessive safety behaviors or avoidance of activities perceived as risky, even when the actual danger is minimal.

Case Example: Sarah checks locks multiple times each night, avoids driving on highways, and constantly worries about family members' safety. She researches every symptom online and assumes worst-case scenarios for minor health concerns.

8. Enmeshment/Undeveloped Self Schema The belief that you cannot survive or be happy without the constant support and involvement of important others. This schema involves excessive emotional involvement with others at the expense of individual identity and autonomy.

People with this schema struggle to differentiate their own feelings and needs from those of others. They may feel empty or directionless when alone and have difficulty making independent decisions.

232

Case Example: Amanda can't make decisions without consulting her best friend and feels anxious when separated from close relationships. She adopts others' interests as her own and struggles to identify her personal preferences and goals.

9. Failure Schema The belief that you have failed or will inevitably fail in areas of achievement relative to peers. This schema involves feeling inadequate in performance areas like career, school, or sports.

This pattern often leads to giving up easily, procrastination, or avoiding challenges to prevent failure. People may underperform despite having adequate abilities due to fear of not meeting expectations.

Case Example: Tom avoids applying for promotions despite excellent performance reviews, believing he would fail in higher-level positions. He procrastinates on important projects and settles for less challenging work to avoid potential failure.

Domain III: Impaired Limits

This domain involves difficulty with self-control, respect for others' rights, and following rules. These schemas often develop when children aren't given appropriate limits or aren't required to tolerate normal frustrations.

10. Grandiosity/Entitlement Schema The belief that you are superior to others and entitled to special rights and privileges. This schema involves difficulty accepting limitations and may include seeking power or control over others.

People with this schema may have difficulty following rules, waiting their turn, or accepting feedback. They often expect special treatment and may become angry when others don't recognize their perceived superiority.

Case Example: Kevin expects immediate service in restaurants and becomes furious when asked to wait. He believes rules don't apply to him and feels justified in cutting lines or demanding exceptions to policies.

11. Insufficient Self-Control/Self-Discipline Schema The difficulty tolerating frustration when trying to achieve goals, along with inability to restrain expression of impulses and emotions. This schema involves poor self-control and difficulty delaying gratification.

This pattern often leads to impulsive behavior, addiction problems, and difficulty completing long-term goals. People may struggle with anger management, spending, eating, or other impulse control issues.

Case Example: Rachel repeatedly starts diet and exercise programs but quits within weeks when progress feels slow. She makes impulsive purchases she can't afford and sends angry emails she later regrets when frustrated at work.

Domain IV: Other-Directedness

This domain includes schemas where focus on others' desires and reactions takes precedence over your own needs. These patterns often develop in families where love and acceptance are conditional on meeting others' needs or expectations.

12. Subjugation Schema The belief that you must submit to others' control because your needs and feelings are not important. This schema involves suppressing your desires to avoid conflict, rejection, or abandonment.

People with this schema often feel angry underneath their compliance but fear expressing disagreement. They may not even recognize their own needs due to chronic focus on pleasing others.

Case Example: Patricia agrees to work overtime every weekend despite wanting time with family, believing that saying no would mark her as selfish and difficult. She suppresses resentment until it explodes in passive-aggressive behavior.

13. Self-Sacrifice Schema The voluntary sacrifice of your own needs to help others, often accompanied by hypersensitivity to others' pain. This schema involves focusing excessively on others' needs while neglecting your own wellbeing.

Unlike subjugation, self-sacrifice is chosen rather than forced, but both patterns result in neglect of personal needs. People may derive identity and worth from helping others while feeling empty and resentful.

Case Example: Mark cancels his vacation to help a colleague with a project, then feels resentful when his sacrifice isn't appreciated. He consistently prioritizes others' needs while his own goals and relationships suffer from neglect.

14. Approval-Seeking/Recognition-Seeking Schema The excessive emphasis on gaining approval and recognition from others at the expense of developing authentic identity. This schema involves basing self-worth on others' opinions and reactions.

People with this schema may be people-pleasers who struggle to express authentic preferences when they differ from others' expectations. They often feel empty and uncertain about their true identity.

Case Example: Jessica changes her opinions based on her audience and feels anxious when others seem displeased with her. She chooses career paths and relationships based on others' approval rather than personal interest or compatibility.

Domain V: Overvigilance and Inhibition

This domain includes schemas that involve excessive control, responsibility, or suppression of emotions and impulses. These patterns often develop in demanding families where performance, duty, and perfectionism are emphasized over spontaneity and pleasure.

15. Negativity/Pessimism Schema The pervasive focus on negative aspects of life while minimizing positive elements. This schema involves chronic worry, vigilance for problems, and pessimistic expectations about outcomes.

People with this schema often feel anxious and hypervigilant, constantly preparing for potential problems. They may have difficulty enjoying positive experiences due to anticipation of future difficulties.

Case Example: Helen focuses on everything that could go wrong with her daughter's wedding instead of enjoying the celebration. She researches worst-case scenarios and creates backup plans for unlikely disasters while missing the joy of the occasion.

16. Emotional Inhibition Schema The excessive inhibition of emotions, spontaneity, and communication to avoid disapproval or losing control. This schema involves suppressing feelings and maintaining rigid control over emotional expression.

This pattern often leads to difficulty with intimacy and authentic self-expression. People may appear calm and controlled while feeling disconnected from their emotional life and others.

Case Example: George maintains emotional distance even with family members, rarely expressing feelings or needs directly. He appears unaffected by stress but feels isolated and struggles to connect meaningfully with others.

17. Unrelenting Standards/Hypercriticalism Schema The belief that you must meet very high standards of performance to avoid criticism. This schema involves perfectionism, rigid rules, and harsh self-criticism when standards aren't met.

People with this schema often work excessively and feel stressed about performance. They may procrastinate due to fear of imperfection or burn out from unsustainable standards.

Case Example: Carol revises work projects endlessly, never feeling satisfied with the quality. She works 70-hour weeks and criticizes herself harshly for minor mistakes while achieving excellent results that she can't appreciate.

18. Punitiveness Schema The belief that people should be harshly punished for mistakes and shortcomings. This schema involves intolerance for errors and quick anger when expectations aren't met.

This pattern affects both self-treatment and relationships with others. People may be highly critical and unforgiving, creating difficult interpersonal dynamics and internal emotional harshness.

Case Example: Dan becomes furious with himself and others for minor mistakes, believing that forgiveness leads to weakness and repeated errors. He holds grudges and expects harsh consequences for any failures or shortcomings.

Recently Added Schemas

19. Approval-Seeking Schema (separated from Recognition-Seeking) The specific focus on gaining approval and avoiding disapproval from others, involving chronic anxiety about others' opinions and reactions.

20. Recognition-Seeking Schema (separated from Approval-Seeking) The drive for attention, admiration, and recognition of achievements, often involving competitive behavior and need for special status.

Understanding Schema Combinations

Most people have multiple schemas that interact to create unique patterns of thinking, feeling, and behaving. Some schemas commonly occur together (like Abandonment and Emotional Deprivation), while others may conflict with each other (like Dependence and Grandiosity). Understanding these interactions helps explain complex psychological presentations and guides treatment planning.

Schemas also vary in intensity from mild to severe, and in pervasiveness from affecting specific life areas to influencing most aspects of functioning. This variation explains why people with the same schemas may have very different presentations and require different therapeutic approaches.

A Foundation for Understanding

These 20 schemas provide the foundation for all schema therapy work, serving as a map for understanding how early experiences continue to influence adult functioning. Each schema represents an understandable adaptation to childhood circumstances that has outlived its usefulness, creating problems in current relationships and life satisfaction.

The goal of schema work isn't eliminating these patterns entirely— they're part of your psychological makeup. Instead, the aim is reducing their intensity and influence while developing healthier responses that serve your current needs and goals more effectively.

Essential Elements for Schema Recognition

- The 20 Early Maladaptive Schemas organize into five domains based on unmet childhood needs
- Each schema includes specific beliefs about self, others, and the world that create predictable patterns
- Schemas vary in intensity and pervasiveness, creating unique individual presentations
- Most people have multiple schemas that interact in complex ways
- Understanding schema definitions provides the foundation for recognition and treatment planning
- Schemas represent understandable adaptations that have outlived their usefulness
- The goal is reducing schema influence rather than complete elimination

Appendix B: Schema Mode Reference Guide

Schema modes represent the emotional states and coping responses that everyone experiences moment to moment throughout their day. Unlike schemas, which are relatively stable traits, modes shift and change based on what triggers you encounter and how you interpret your experiences[84]. Understanding modes helps you recognize which part of yourself is active at any given time and provides tools for accessing healthier responses to challenging situations.

The mode concept acknowledges that human beings are complex, with different parts that serve different functions. Sometimes your Vulnerable Child mode is active, feeling small and scared in response to criticism. Other times your Demanding Parent mode takes charge, pushing yourself and others toward impossible standards. The goal of mode work is helping your Healthy Adult mode serve as the wise coordinator of all these different parts.

Child Modes

Child modes represent the emotional, spontaneous, and need-based aspects of personality. These modes carry both wounds from childhood and the capacity for joy, creativity, and authentic expression. Understanding child modes helps you respond to these parts with appropriate care rather than criticism or suppression.

Vulnerable Child Mode This mode carries the core emotional wounds and unmet needs from childhood. When active, you feel small, hurt, lonely, afraid, or sad—much like you did as a child facing overwhelming circumstances. This mode needs comfort, validation, and protection rather than harsh treatment or demands for immediate strength.

The Vulnerable Child holds your deepest needs for love, safety, and acceptance. While it can feel overwhelming when activated, this mode also contains your capacity for emotional connection and authentic feeling. Learning to nurture rather than suppress this mode is essential for emotional healing.

Case Example: When Lisa's supervisor gives feedback on her presentation, her Vulnerable Child mode activates, leaving her feeling eight years old and devastated by criticism. She wants to hide under her desk and cry, feeling like the inadequate child who could never please her critical father.

Angry Child Mode This mode expresses the rage and protest about unmet needs and unfair treatment. When active, you may feel furious, rebellious, or defiant—expressing the anger that couldn't be safely expressed during childhood. This mode often emerges when the Vulnerable Child's needs are dismissed or ignored.

The Angry Child mode serves an important function by recognizing injustice and advocating for fair treatment. However, it may express anger in ways that are inappropriate for adult situations, requiring guidance from the Healthy Adult mode about effective expression.

Case Example: When Tom's wife suggests he help more with household chores, his Angry Child mode explodes with rage about being criticized and controlled. He feels like the rebellious teenager whose parents demanded perfection while never acknowledging his efforts or contributions.

Impulsive Child Mode This mode seeks immediate gratification and acts on desires without considering consequences. When active, you may engage in impulsive behaviors like overspending, overeating, substance use, or sexual acting out. This mode wants what it wants when it wants it.

The Impulsive Child often emerges when emotional needs aren't being met through healthy channels. While this mode can create problems through poor impulse control, it also contains your capacity for spontaneity, pleasure, and living in the moment.

Case Example: After a stressful week at work, Jennifer's Impulsive Child mode takes over during a shopping trip, leading her to purchase expensive clothes she doesn't need and can't afford. She feels temporary relief but later faces guilt and financial stress.

Happy Child Mode This mode represents your capacity for joy, wonder, creativity, and playfulness. When active, you feel spontaneous, excited, and fully engaged with life. This mode emerges when you feel safe, loved, and free to express your authentic self without fear of criticism or rejection.

The Happy Child mode is the goal of much therapeutic work—not constant happiness, but the ability to access joy and spontaneity when circumstances allow. This mode often becomes suppressed when life feels too dangerous or demanding for playfulness.

Case Example: During a weekend camping trip with close friends, David's Happy Child mode emerges as he laughs freely, tells stories, and feels genuinely connected and joyful. He experiences the carefree spirit that was rarely safe to express during his controlled childhood.

Dysfunctional Parent Modes

Parent modes represent internalized voices and messages from childhood authority figures. These modes can be helpful when they provide appropriate guidance and standards, but become problematic when they're harsh, demanding, or critical in ways that damage self-esteem and wellbeing.

Punitive Parent Mode This mode delivers harsh criticism, punishment, and blame for mistakes or perceived shortcomings. When active, you may engage in brutal self-attack, feeling that you deserve punishment for not being perfect. This mode often uses language like "should," "must," and "always/never."

The Punitive Parent mode typically developed from harsh, critical, or abusive treatment during childhood. While it may motivate behavior through fear, it creates shame and self-hatred that ultimately interfere with healthy functioning and self-improvement.

Case Example: When Sandra makes a minor error in a work email, her Punitive Parent mode launches a vicious internal attack: "You're so careless and stupid. Everyone will think you're incompetent. You

241

don't deserve this job and you'll probably get fired for being such an idiot."

Demanding Parent Mode This mode pushes relentlessly toward achievement, perfectionism, and meeting others' expectations. When active, you may feel driven to work constantly, achieve at impossible levels, and sacrifice personal needs for productivity or approval. This mode often creates chronic stress and burnout.

The Demanding Parent often developed in families where love was conditional on performance or achievement. While it can motivate success, it creates an internal taskmaster that's never satisfied and doesn't allow for rest or self-compassion.

Case Example: Robert's Demanding Parent mode won't let him enjoy his promotion because there's always more to achieve. It pushes him to work 80-hour weeks and criticizes any time spent on personal interests as laziness or lack of ambition.

Coping Modes

Coping modes represent the strategies you developed to manage overwhelming emotions and difficult life circumstances. While these modes served important protective functions, they often create problems in current relationships and life satisfaction when used excessively.

Compliant Surrenderer Mode This mode submits to others' demands and gives up trying to get your own needs met. When active, you may feel resigned, hopeless, and passive, going along with others' wishes while suppressing your own preferences and desires.

The Compliant Surrenderer often developed when resistance to others' demands felt dangerous or futile. While it can prevent conflict in the short term, it leads to resentment and loss of personal identity over time.

Case Example: Maria's Compliant Surrenderer mode automatically agrees when her mother demands she spend every holiday at the family home, despite wanting to create new traditions with her own family. She feels powerless to resist and resigned to always doing what others expect.

Detached Protector Mode This mode creates emotional distance and numbness to avoid being hurt by others. When active, you may feel disconnected, empty, or like you're going through the motions of life without genuine engagement. This mode protects against emotional pain by preventing emotional connection.

The Detached Protector typically developed when emotions felt too dangerous or overwhelming to experience fully. While it provides protection from pain, it also cuts you off from positive emotions and meaningful relationships.

Case Example: During his divorce proceedings, Michael's Detached Protector mode allows him to function at work and handle legal meetings, but he feels like he's watching his life from behind glass, unable to connect with his emotions or other people.

Overcompensator Mode This mode fights against schemas by acting in the opposite direction, often to an extreme degree. When active, you may become controlling, aggressive, narcissistic, or competitive to avoid feeling vulnerable or inadequate. This mode tries to prove that schema fears aren't true.

The Overcompensator often develops when schemas feel too painful to acknowledge directly. While it can create external success and prevent others from seeing vulnerability, it often damages relationships and prevents authentic self-expression.

Case Example: To combat his Defectiveness schema, James's Overcompensator mode makes him act superior and critical toward others, constantly proving his intelligence and competence while secretly feeling fraudulent and inadequate underneath the performance.

Healthy Adult Mode

The Healthy Adult mode represents your wise, balanced, and mature self that can handle life's challenges with flexibility and skill. This mode can nurture your Child modes, set appropriate limits on Parent modes, and choose when coping modes are helpful versus harmful.

Characteristics of Healthy Adult Mode

- Emotional regulation without suppression or overwhelming reactivity
- Realistic thinking that considers multiple perspectives and evidence
- Appropriate assertiveness that respects both your needs and others' rights
- Self-compassion that acknowledges mistakes without harsh self-attack
- Relationship skills that allow for both intimacy and healthy boundaries
- Goal-directed behavior that balances achievement with self-care
- Present-moment awareness that prevents being overwhelmed by past or future concerns

Developing Healthy Adult Mode The Healthy Adult mode strengthens through practice and conscious cultivation. Unlike other modes that often activate automatically, the Healthy Adult typically requires intentional access, especially during stressful situations when other modes may feel more familiar.

Case Example: When Patricia receives criticism from her supervisor, her Healthy Adult mode helps her listen to the feedback without becoming overwhelmed (avoiding Vulnerable Child activation), respond professionally without attacking back (avoiding Angry Child), and consider the validity of the feedback while maintaining self-respect (avoiding both Compliant Surrenderer and Overcompensator responses).

Mode Interactions and Sequences

Modes rarely operate in isolation—they typically activate in predictable sequences and combinations that create your unique emotional and behavioral patterns. Understanding these interactions helps you recognize mode patterns and intervene more effectively.

Common Mode Sequences:

- Vulnerable Child activation often triggers Demanding Parent criticism, leading to Detached Protector withdrawal
- Angry Child expression may activate Punitive Parent self-attack, resulting in Compliant Surrenderer submission
- Impulsive Child behavior frequently leads to Demanding Parent demands for control and perfection

Mode Conflicts: Some modes directly oppose each other, creating internal battles that can feel confusing and exhausting. The Healthy Adult mode can mediate these conflicts by understanding what each mode needs and finding balanced solutions.

Mode Work in Daily Life

Effective mode work involves recognizing which mode is active, understanding what triggered the activation, and choosing how to respond based on your current circumstances rather than automatic patterns. This creates flexibility and choice in emotional responses.

Mode Recognition Skills:

- Notice changes in your emotional state, body language, and internal voice
- Identify which mode's language and concerns match your current experience
- Recognize environmental or interpersonal triggers that activate specific modes
- Observe mode transitions and what causes them to shift

Mode Response Skills:

- Validate each mode's concerns while choosing appropriate responses
- Access your Healthy Adult mode during challenging situations
- Provide appropriate care for Child modes without letting them control decisions
- Set limits on dysfunctional Parent modes while accessing their helpful guidance
- Use coping modes consciously rather than automatically

Working with Different Modes

Each mode requires different responses and interventions. Child modes need nurturing and validation, Parent modes need limits and perspective, coping modes need appreciation for their protective function along with guidance about appropriate use, and the Healthy Adult mode needs strengthening and practice.

Understanding modes provides a framework for internal self-care that honors all parts of yourself while allowing your wisest self to guide important decisions and responses. This internal democracy, led by the Healthy Adult, creates emotional health and relationship satisfaction.

Essential Elements for Mode Work

- Schema modes represent temporary emotional states rather than permanent personality traits
- Child modes carry both wounds and capacities that need nurturing rather than suppression
- Parent modes provide both helpful guidance and harmful criticism that require conscious evaluation
- Coping modes serve protective functions that may become problematic when overused
- The Healthy Adult mode can coordinate all other modes while providing wise leadership

- Mode recognition skills help identify which part of you is active at any given moment
- Mode work creates emotional flexibility and conscious choice rather than automatic reactivity

Appendix C: Troubleshooting Common Challenges in Schema Work

Schema therapy, like any deep psychological work, presents predictable challenges that can slow progress or create temporary setbacks. Understanding these common obstacles helps both therapists and clients navigate difficulties with realistic expectations and effective strategies[85]. Most challenges in schema work stem from the very patterns the therapy aims to change—schemas resist modification because they feel protective and familiar, even when they create problems.

The troubleshooting approach recognizes that challenges are normal parts of the healing process rather than signs of failure or inadequacy. Each obstacle provides information about schema patterns and opportunities to practice new responses in real-time therapeutic situations. This appendix provides specific guidance for addressing the most frequent challenges encountered in schema therapy work.

Resistance to Schema Identification

Many clients initially resist recognizing or accepting their schema patterns, particularly when schemas feel shameful or threaten their self-concept. This resistance often reflects schema patterns themselves—the Defectiveness schema may insist that having problems means you're fundamentally flawed, while the Self-Reliance schema may view needing help as weakness.

Common Manifestations of Resistance:

- Intellectual understanding without emotional connection to schema patterns
- Minimizing the impact of childhood experiences on current functioning
- Focusing on external factors rather than internal patterns
- Arguing with assessment results or therapeutic interpretations
- Frequent missed appointments or homework non-compliance

Case Example: Mark's Defensive Intellectualization Mark, a 42-year-old attorney, approached schema therapy like a legal case, analyzing concepts intellectually while avoiding emotional connection to his patterns. When presented with evidence of his Unrelenting Standards schema, he argued that high standards were professional requirements rather than problematic patterns.

Mark's resistance served multiple functions: protecting his professional identity, avoiding shame about childhood experiences with critical parents, and maintaining control through intellectual analysis. His schema insisted that accepting "problems" would confirm his inadequacy and threaten his carefully constructed self-image.

Troubleshooting Strategies for Resistance:

- Normalize resistance as protective and understandable rather than problematic
- Explore what schemas might be driving the resistance itself
- Use collaborative rather than confrontational approaches to schema identification
- Provide psychoeducation about how schemas develop as smart adaptations
- Start with less threatening schemas before addressing core patterns
- Use client's language and metaphors rather than clinical terminology

Overwhelming Emotional Activation

Some clients become flooded with emotions during schema work, particularly when processing traumatic memories or deep wounds. This activation can feel dangerous and may trigger avoidance or premature termination of therapy. The challenge involves allowing emotional processing while maintaining safety and stability.

Signs of Overwhelming Activation:

- Dissociation or disconnection during sessions
- Severe emotional reactions that persist between sessions
- Increase in self-destructive behaviors or crisis episodes
- Inability to function normally after therapy sessions
- Strong urges to avoid therapy or end treatment

Case Example: Sarah's Abandonment Flooding Sarah, a 28-year-old teacher, became overwhelmed during imagery work addressing her Abandonment schema. Accessing childhood memories of her father's departure triggered such intense panic that she couldn't sleep for days and called in sick to work. She wanted to quit therapy to avoid further emotional pain.

Sarah's flooding reflected her nervous system's attempt to protect her from retraumatization, but her all-or-nothing response (either avoid completely or dive too deep) was characteristic of her schema patterns. Her emotional system hadn't learned to tolerate moderate levels of distress without becoming overwhelmed.

Troubleshooting Strategies for Emotional Overwhelm:

- Slow down the pace of therapy and build stabilization skills first
- Teach grounding and emotional regulation techniques before processing work
- Use titrated exposure rather than full-intensity emotional processing
- Provide between-session support and crisis planning
- Consider medication consultation for severe emotional dysregulation
- Focus on building distress tolerance before deeper trauma work

Lack of Progress or Plateau Periods

Some clients feel stuck or discouraged when progress feels slow or imperceptible. Schema change happens gradually, and improvement often occurs in ways that clients don't immediately recognize. Plateau periods are normal parts of healing that may reflect integration time or preparation for the next growth phase.

Common Expressions of Feeling Stuck:

- "Nothing is changing despite months of therapy"
- "I understand my schemas but still react the same way"
- "Other people seem to progress faster than I do"
- "Maybe I'm just too damaged/old/stubborn to change"
- "This therapy isn't working for me"

Case Example: Jennifer's Hidden Progress Jennifer, a 35-year-old nurse, felt discouraged after six months of schema work because she still felt anxious in relationships and struggled with people-pleasing. She hadn't noticed that her anxiety episodes were shorter and less intense, she was setting small boundaries consistently, and others commented on her increased assertiveness.

Jennifer's Self-Sacrifice schema made her focus on what she wasn't giving others rather than recognizing her own growth. Her Unrelenting Standards schema demanded rapid, dramatic change rather than appreciating gradual improvement. Her schemas were actually preventing her from recognizing the progress she was making.

Troubleshooting Strategies for Plateau Periods:

- Use objective measures to track progress that may not be subjectively obvious
- Normalize plateau periods as necessary integration and consolidation time
- Explore whether schemas are preventing recognition of actual progress
- Adjust expectations about the pace and nature of schema change
- Celebrate small improvements rather than waiting for dramatic breakthroughs
- Consider whether therapy approach needs modification for individual needs

251

Difficulty Accessing Emotions

Some clients struggle to connect with their emotional experience, particularly those with strong Emotional Inhibition schemas or histories of trauma that required emotional suppression for survival. This emotional disconnection can make schema work feel purely intellectual without the emotional processing necessary for deep change.

Signs of Emotional Disconnection:

- Describing events without corresponding emotional reactions
- Intellectualizing feelings rather than experiencing them
- Difficulty identifying or naming emotions
- Physical symptoms without emotional awareness
- Feeling "numb" or "empty" most of the time

Case Example: Robert's Emotional Wall Robert, a 39-year-old engineer, could analyze his schemas intellectually but couldn't access the emotions connected to his childhood experiences. He described severe emotional neglect in a matter-of-fact tone while showing no emotional response to clearly painful memories.

Robert's emotional disconnection had protected him through a childhood where emotions were dangerous—expressing needs led to criticism, showing pain brought more abuse, and emotional expression was seen as weakness. His survival had depended on emotional shutdown, but this protection now prevented the emotional connection necessary for healing.

Troubleshooting Strategies for Emotional Disconnection:

- Start with body awareness and physical sensations before targeting emotions
- Use experiential techniques like imagery and chair work to bypass intellectual defenses
- Explore the protective function of emotional disconnection before trying to change it

- Practice identifying and naming emotions in low-stakes situations
- Address trauma and safety issues that may require emotional numbing
- Consider somatic therapies or bodywork as adjuncts to schema therapy

Relationship Difficulties with the Therapist

Schema patterns often emerge in the therapeutic relationship itself, creating challenges that can either derail therapy or provide powerful opportunities for healing. Common issues include testing behaviors, boundary violations, excessive dependency, or recreating familiar dysfunctional dynamics.

Common Therapeutic Relationship Challenges:

- Testing therapist's commitment through difficult behaviors
- Becoming overly dependent on therapist for emotional regulation
- Expecting rejection or abandonment from therapist
- Feeling criticized or judged during feedback or interventions
- Recreating family dynamics with therapist in parental role

Case Example: Maria's Abandonment Testing Maria repeatedly tested her therapist's commitment by canceling sessions last-minute, arriving late, or engaging in crisis behaviors before important sessions. She simultaneously craved her therapist's care and tried to prove that the therapist would eventually reject her like others had.

Maria's testing served multiple functions: confirming her Abandonment schema's predictions, maintaining familiar relationship patterns, and protecting herself from hoped-for but feared emotional connection. Her behaviors created the very rejection she feared while preventing the therapeutic relationship from contradicting her schema.

Troubleshooting Strategies for Relationship Difficulties:

- Address therapeutic relationship issues directly and collaboratively
- Use relationship patterns as live examples of schema activation
- Maintain appropriate boundaries while providing consistent care
- Explore client's expectations and fears about the therapeutic relationship
- Process relationship ruptures as opportunities for corrective experiences
- Consider consultation or supervision for complex relationship dynamics

Homework Non-Compliance

Many clients struggle with completing between-session assignments, which can slow progress and create therapy obstacles. Non-compliance often reflects schema patterns themselves—perfectionism may prevent starting assignments that might be done imperfectly, while Emotional Deprivation schemas may view homework as additional demands rather than self-care.

Common Reasons for Non-Compliance:

- Assignments feel too difficult or overwhelming
- Perfectionism prevents starting tasks that might be done imperfectly
- Assignments trigger schema activation or emotional distress
- Lack of understanding about assignment purpose or instructions
- Life circumstances prevent consistent homework completion

Case Example: David's Perfectionist Paralysis David consistently failed to complete thought records and behavioral experiments, despite expressing commitment to therapy goals. His Unrelenting Standards schema made him spend hours trying to complete assignments perfectly, leading to frustration and eventual abandonment of the tasks.

David's non-compliance reflected his schema patterns directly—he couldn't tolerate doing assignments imperfectly, but perfectionist completion was so time-consuming that he couldn't sustain the effort. His homework difficulties became a direct example of how his schemas interfered with his goals.

Troubleshooting Strategies for Homework Issues:

- Collaborate on assignment design to ensure appropriateness and feasibility
- Explore what schemas might be interfering with homework completion
- Start with very brief, simple assignments to build success experiences
- Address perfectionism or other schemas that create homework obstacles
- Provide flexibility and alternatives when life circumstances interfere
- Use homework difficulties as therapeutic material rather than just compliance issues

Crisis and Safety Concerns

Some clients experience crisis episodes during schema work, particularly when processing trauma or when life stressors activate multiple schemas simultaneously. While crises can provide therapeutic opportunities, they require careful management to maintain safety while supporting continued growth.

Types of Crisis Situations:

- Suicidal ideation or self-harm behaviors
- Severe anxiety or panic episodes
- Relationship crises that threaten important connections
- Work or academic performance problems
- Substance use or other behavioral acting out

Crisis Management Strategies:

- Develop comprehensive safety plans before crises occur
- Maintain clear boundaries about therapist availability and emergency procedures
- Coordinate with other providers (psychiatrists, primary care, etc.) as needed
- Use crisis episodes as opportunities to practice new coping skills
- Address underlying schemas that may be contributing to crisis vulnerability
- Consider intensive outpatient or inpatient treatment for severe safety concerns

Building Resilience Through Challenges

The challenges encountered in schema work often provide the most powerful opportunities for growth and healing. Each obstacle reveals schema patterns in action and creates chances to practice new responses in real-time. Successful navigation of therapy challenges builds confidence and resilience that transfer to other life areas.

The key to effective troubleshooting involves viewing challenges as information rather than failures, maintaining realistic expectations about the pace of change, and using obstacles as opportunities to deepen understanding and practice new skills. With appropriate support and intervention, most therapy challenges can be resolved in ways that actually strengthen the therapeutic work.

Essential Elements for Challenge Navigation

- Resistance to schema identification often reflects schema patterns themselves and requires gentle, collaborative exploration
- Overwhelming emotional activation needs careful pacing and stabilization before deeper processing work
- Plateau periods are normal parts of healing that may reflect necessary integration time rather than lack of progress
- Emotional disconnection serves protective functions that must be understood before attempting to increase emotional access

- Therapeutic relationship difficulties provide opportunities for corrective experiences when handled skillfully
- Homework non-compliance often reflects schema interference rather than lack of motivation
- Crisis situations require safety planning and may accelerate therapeutic progress when managed appropriately

Appendix D: Integration with Other Therapeutic Modalities

Schema Therapy's integrative foundation makes it naturally compatible with other evidence-based therapeutic approaches. Rather than viewing different therapies as competing methodologies, skilled clinicians can combine Schema Therapy with complementary modalities to address complex presentations and maximize therapeutic effectiveness[86]. This integration requires understanding how different approaches work together synergistically rather than simply adding techniques without theoretical coherence.

The integration process involves identifying which therapeutic modalities address aspects of client functioning that Schema Therapy might not fully target, while ensuring that combined approaches support rather than contradict each other. Effective integration maintains the core principles of each modality while creating a coherent treatment plan that serves the client's unique needs and circumstances.

Cognitive-Behavioral Therapy Integration

CBT integration with Schema Therapy represents the most natural combination, given Schema Therapy's cognitive-behavioral foundations. Traditional CBT focuses on current symptoms and surface-level cognitions, while Schema Therapy addresses deeper belief systems and childhood origins. Together, they provide both immediate symptom relief and long-term pattern change.

Complementary Strengths:

- CBT provides structured symptom management techniques
- Schema Therapy addresses underlying patterns that maintain symptoms
- CBT offers specific tools for anxiety, depression, and behavioral problems

258

- Schema Therapy explains why CBT techniques may not work for some clients
- Combined approach addresses both current functioning and developmental origins

Case Example: Integrated Treatment for Rebecca's Anxiety

Rebecca, a 31-year-old teacher, presented with panic disorder and social anxiety that hadn't responded adequately to standard CBT. Integration of Schema Therapy revealed underlying Vulnerability to Harm and Social Isolation schemas that maintained her anxiety despite learning CBT coping skills.

The integrated treatment combined CBT's anxiety management techniques with Schema Therapy's exploration of childhood origins. Rebecca learned breathing exercises and exposure techniques from CBT while using Schema Therapy to address her core beliefs about danger and social rejection. The CBT tools provided immediate relief while Schema work addressed why her anxiety kept returning.

The integration was particularly effective because CBT's structured approach appealed to Rebecca's need for concrete tools, while Schema Therapy's developmental focus helped her understand why she needed these tools in the first place. Neither approach alone would have been as effective as their thoughtful combination.

Integration Guidelines for CBT:

- Use CBT techniques for immediate symptom management while Schema work addresses underlying patterns
- Apply Schema understanding to explain CBT homework resistance or technique ineffectiveness
- Modify CBT interventions based on client's schema patterns and coping styles
- Use Schema concepts to understand why certain CBT techniques work better for different clients
- Combine CBT's present-focus with Schema Therapy's developmental perspective

Trauma Therapy Integration

Many clients with significant schemas have trauma histories that require specialized intervention. Schema Therapy can be enhanced by trauma-specific approaches like EMDR, Cognitive Processing Therapy, or Trauma-Focused CBT that address specific traumatic incidents while Schema work heals the broader patterns that developed in response.

Complementary Functions:

- Trauma therapies address specific incidents and PTSD symptoms
- Schema Therapy addresses broader patterns and relationship impacts
- Trauma work can reduce schema intensity by healing underlying wounds
- Schema work provides context for understanding trauma's ongoing impact
- Combined approaches address both specific memories and general life patterns

Case Example: Combined EMDR and Schema Therapy for Michael Michael, a 35-year-old veteran, presented with complex PTSD from both combat trauma and childhood abuse. EMDR effectively processed specific traumatic memories, but his Mistrust and Vulnerability schemas continued creating relationship difficulties and chronic hypervigilance.

The integrated treatment used EMDR to process specific traumatic incidents while Schema Therapy addressed the broader patterns of mistrust and fear that affected all his relationships. EMDR reduced the emotional charge of particular memories while Schema work helped Michael understand how trauma had shaped his entire approach to relationships and safety.

The combination was essential because EMDR alone didn't address Michael's relationship schemas, while Schema Therapy alone might not have provided sufficient trauma processing. Together, they addressed both specific traumatic memories and general life patterns that trauma had created.

Integration Guidelines for Trauma Therapy:

- Use trauma-specific techniques for PTSD symptoms while Schema work addresses broader patterns
- Ensure adequate stabilization before combining intensive trauma processing with schema work
- Coordinate trauma processing with schema healing to prevent retraumatization
- Use Schema understanding to predict which trauma interventions will be most effective
- Address both specific traumatic incidents and general schema patterns that trauma created

Mindfulness-Based Interventions

Mindfulness approaches like MBSR, MBCT, or ACT complement Schema Therapy by providing present-moment awareness tools that help clients observe schema activation without being overwhelmed by it. Mindfulness skills support the Healthy Adult mode while creating space between schema triggers and automatic responses.

Complementary Benefits:

- Mindfulness provides tools for observing schemas without being controlled by them
- Schema Therapy explains what to do with schema patterns once you're aware of them
- Mindfulness builds emotional regulation capacity needed for schema work
- Schema work provides context for understanding why mindfulness is difficult
- Combined approaches address both awareness and action components of change

Case Example: Mindfulness-Enhanced Schema Work for Patricia
Patricia, a 33-year-old social worker, struggled with Self-Sacrifice schemas that created chronic overwhelm and resentment. Adding mindfulness practices to her Schema Therapy helped her notice when she was automatically saying yes to requests before schema patterns took control.

The mindfulness component taught Patricia to pause and observe her automatic reactions, creating space for conscious choice about how to respond. Schema Therapy provided understanding of why certain situations triggered automatic helping behaviors and offered alternative responses that honored both her caring nature and personal needs.

The integration was particularly powerful because mindfulness helped Patricia catch schema activation early, while Schema work gave her specific tools for responding differently once she noticed the patterns. Neither approach alone would have provided both the awareness and action components she needed.

Integration Guidelines for Mindfulness:

- Use mindfulness skills to create space between schema activation and automatic responses
- Apply Schema understanding to explain why mindfulness practice is difficult
- Combine mindfulness awareness with Schema Therapy action strategies
- Use mindfulness to strengthen the Healthy Adult mode's capacity for conscious choice
- Integrate mindfulness practices into daily schema maintenance routines

Attachment-Based Therapies

Attachment-focused approaches like Emotionally Focused Therapy share significant overlap with Schema Therapy's focus on early relationships and their ongoing impact. Integration can be particularly powerful for couples work, where individual schemas create relationship patterns that require both individual and systemic intervention.

Overlapping Elements:

- Both approaches focus on early attachment experiences and their ongoing impact
- Attachment therapy addresses relationship patterns while Schema work addresses individual patterns
- Combined approaches can address both partners' schemas and their interaction patterns
- Attachment focus complements Schema Therapy's relationship emphasis
- Integration provides both individual healing and relationship improvement

Case Example: Couples Schema Therapy with EFT Integration
David and Sarah, married for eight years, struggled with recurring conflicts that reflected their individual schemas. David's Emotional Deprivation schema made him withdraw during conflicts, while Sarah's Abandonment schema made her pursue and demand connection, creating a pursue-withdraw cycle.

The integrated treatment combined individual Schema work to address each partner's patterns with EFT techniques to improve their communication and connection. Schema work helped each partner understand their own and their partner's reactions, while EFT provided tools for breaking negative cycles and creating positive interactions.

The integration was essential because individual Schema work alone didn't address their interaction patterns, while couples work alone didn't address the individual schemas that fueled their conflicts. Together, they created both individual healing and relationship improvement.

Integration Guidelines for Attachment Therapy:

- Address individual schemas that contribute to relationship patterns
- Use attachment understanding to inform Schema work priorities
- Combine individual schema healing with relationship skill building
- Apply Schema concepts to understand attachment injuries and their repair
- Integrate Schema maintenance with ongoing relationship practices

Psychodynamic Integration

Psychodynamic approaches can complement Schema Therapy by providing additional insight into unconscious patterns and defense mechanisms. While Schema Therapy is more structured and present-focused, psychodynamic understanding can deepen comprehension of how schemas developed and continue to operate outside conscious awareness.

Complementary Perspectives:

- Psychodynamic work explores unconscious patterns while Schema work makes patterns conscious
- Defense mechanism understanding enhances comprehension of coping modes
- Transference analysis can illuminate schema patterns in therapeutic relationships
- Psychodynamic insight can deepen understanding of schema origins
- Schema structure can organize psychodynamic insights into actionable frameworks

Integration Considerations:

- Balance insight-oriented work with Schema Therapy's action-focused approach

- Use psychodynamic understanding to inform Schema conceptualization
- Apply Schema frameworks to organize psychodynamic insights
- Maintain focus on current functioning while exploring unconscious patterns
- Integrate unconscious awareness with conscious schema change efforts

Family and Systemic Approaches

Family therapy integration recognizes that schemas often develop and are maintained within family systems. Individual Schema work can be enhanced by family interventions that address systemic patterns, while family therapy can benefit from Schema understanding of individual family members' patterns.

Systemic Considerations:

- Individual schemas affect family functioning and vice versa
- Family patterns often reinforce individual schemas across generations
- Schema understanding can guide family intervention strategies
- Family work can support individual schema healing
- Integration addresses both individual and systemic change needs

Creating Coherent Integration

Successful integration requires maintaining theoretical coherence while adapting techniques to individual needs. The process involves understanding how different approaches complement each other, timing interventions appropriately, and ensuring that combined treatments support rather than confuse clients.

Integration Principles:

- Maintain coherent theoretical framework while incorporating diverse techniques
- Sequence interventions based on client readiness and therapeutic phase
- Explain integration rationale to clients to maintain collaboration
- Monitor for technique overload or theoretical confusion
- Adapt integration based on client response and treatment progress

A Unified Approach to Healing

Effective integration transforms Schema Therapy from a single modality into a comprehensive framework that can incorporate the best elements of multiple therapeutic approaches. This flexibility allows for personalized treatment that addresses complex presentations while maintaining theoretical coherence and clinical effectiveness.

The goal of integration isn't using every available technique, but rather thoughtfully combining approaches that address different aspects of client functioning in mutually supportive ways. When done skillfully, integration creates treatment that is more effective than any single modality could achieve alone.

Essential Elements for Therapeutic Integration

- CBT integration provides immediate symptom relief while Schema work addresses underlying patterns
- Trauma therapy combination addresses specific incidents alongside broader schema patterns
- Mindfulness approaches create awareness space that supports conscious schema responses
- Attachment-based therapies complement Schema work's relationship focus with systemic interventions
- Psychodynamic integration deepens understanding of unconscious schema patterns

- Family therapy addresses systemic factors that maintain individual schemas
- Effective integration maintains theoretical coherence while personalizing treatment approaches

Appendix E: Resources for Further Learning and Professional Development

Professional competence in Schema Therapy requires ongoing learning, practice, and supervision beyond initial training. The field continues growing through research, clinical innovation, and international collaboration, creating rich opportunities for continued development[87]. This appendix provides guidance for therapists seeking to deepen their Schema Therapy knowledge and skills while maintaining ethical practice standards and professional growth.

The learning process in Schema Therapy involves both theoretical understanding and experiential practice. Unlike purely cognitive therapies, Schema work requires therapists to understand their own schema patterns and develop the emotional skills necessary for effective experiential interventions. This personal and professional development happens through multiple channels that support both competence and self-awareness.

Professional Training and Certification

The International Society of Schema Therapy (ISST) provides the primary credentialing structure for Schema Therapy training and certification. Their multi-level training model ensures systematic skill development while maintaining quality standards across international training programs.

ISST Training Levels:

Level 1 - Introduction to Schema Therapy provides foundational knowledge about schema theory, assessment methods, and basic intervention techniques. This 32-hour training introduces core concepts and prepares participants for further specialized training. Level 1 is appropriate for mental health professionals seeking basic Schema Therapy knowledge.

Level 2 - Schema Therapy Skills focuses on practical application of Schema Therapy techniques through experiential learning and case discussion. This 32-hour training emphasizes skill development in cognitive, experiential, and behavioral interventions. Participants practice techniques and receive feedback on their developing competence.

Level 3 - Advanced Schema Therapy addresses complex clinical presentations, specialized populations, and advanced intervention techniques. This training requires completion of previous levels and focuses on treating severe personality disorders, trauma-related schemas, and difficult clinical challenges.

Certification Requirements include completed training hours, supervised clinical practice, case presentation, and written examination. Certification demonstrates competence in Schema Therapy practice and qualifies therapists for advanced training and supervision roles.

Case Example: Dr. Anderson's Professional Development Journey Dr. Anderson, a licensed psychologist with 10 years of general therapy experience, pursued Schema Therapy training to better serve clients with personality disorders and treatment-resistant conditions. She completed Level 1 training and immediately noticed improvements in her case conceptualization skills and treatment planning.

Level 2 training provided hands-on practice with techniques like chair work and imagery rescripting, helping Dr. Anderson develop confidence in experiential interventions. She particularly benefited from practicing these techniques herself during training, gaining understanding of their emotional impact and therapeutic potential.

Advanced training and certification required Dr. Anderson to demonstrate competence through supervised cases and examination. This process deepened her understanding while ensuring she could practice Schema Therapy safely and effectively with complex clients.

Essential Reading and Literature

Schema Therapy literature spans foundational texts, research articles, specialized applications, and ongoing developments in the field. Building a solid knowledge base requires engaging with both classic works and current innovations.

Foundational Texts:

"Schema Therapy: A Practitioner's Guide" by Young, Klosko, and Weishaar remains the definitive clinical manual for Schema Therapy practice. This text provides theoretical foundations, assessment procedures, and intervention techniques with detailed case examples and practical guidance.

"Reinventing Your Life" by Young and Klosko offers the client-focused perspective on Schema Therapy, providing accessible explanations of schema concepts and self-help strategies. This book helps therapists understand how to explain concepts to clients and provides homework resources.

"Schema Therapy: Distinctive Features" by Rafaeli, Bernstein, and Young presents Schema Therapy's unique elements and distinguishing characteristics compared to other therapeutic approaches. This concise text helps understand what makes Schema Therapy different and effective.

Specialized Applications:

Literature addressing specific populations includes texts on Schema Therapy for borderline personality disorder, eating disorders, forensic populations, couples therapy, and group applications. These specialized resources provide adapted techniques and considerations for different client presentations.

Research Literature:

Current research appears in journals like Journal of Behavior Therapy and Experimental Psychiatry, Cognitive Therapy and Research, and Clinical Psychology Review. Regular review of research literature keeps practitioners current with effectiveness studies, treatment innovations, and theoretical developments.

Supervision and Consultation

Effective Schema Therapy requires ongoing supervision and consultation, particularly during skill development phases. The complexity of schema work and potential for client destabilization make professional support essential for safe and effective practice.

Types of Professional Support:

Individual Supervision provides personalized guidance on specific cases, technique development, and professional growth. Schema Therapy supervision often includes review of session videos, case conceptualization development, and skills practice.

Group Consultation offers peer learning opportunities and diverse perspectives on challenging cases. Group formats provide cost-effective supervision while building professional community among Schema Therapy practitioners.

Case Consultation addresses specific client situations that require specialized expertise or complex decision-making. Consultation may focus on diagnosis, treatment planning, crisis management, or ethical considerations.

Case Example: Managing Complex Trauma in Schema Work Dr. Martinez consulted with a Schema Therapy expert about a client with severe childhood trauma who was becoming destabilized during imagery work. The consultation helped Dr. Martinez modify her approach to provide better stabilization while continuing therapeutic progress.

The consultant recommended slowing the pace of imagery work, building additional emotional regulation skills, and coordinating with the client's psychiatrist about medication support. This guidance prevented treatment crisis while maintaining therapeutic momentum.

Professional Organizations and Networks

Professional organizations provide continuing education opportunities, networking, and resources for ongoing development in Schema Therapy practice.

International Society of Schema Therapy (ISST) serves as the primary professional organization for Schema Therapy practitioners worldwide. ISST provides training standards, certification processes, annual conferences, and professional resources.

Regional Schema Therapy Organizations exist in many countries and regions, providing local training opportunities, consultation networks, and professional support. These organizations often adapt Schema Therapy training to local cultural and professional contexts.

Professional Conferences offer intensive learning opportunities, networking, and exposure to latest developments in Schema Therapy research and practice. Annual conferences provide workshops, research presentations, and professional development opportunities.

Personal Therapy and Self-Awareness

Schema Therapy practitioners benefit from understanding their own schema patterns and how these might affect their therapeutic work. Personal therapy isn't required for practice but is strongly recommended for professional and personal development.

Benefits of Personal Schema Work:

Understanding your own schemas helps recognize when client patterns might trigger personal reactions. Schema Therapy work can be emotionally intense, and therapist self-awareness prevents personal issues from interfering with client care.

Personal schema work also provides experiential understanding of therapeutic techniques. Having experienced chair work, imagery rescripting, or schema dialogue personally gives therapists authentic appreciation for these interventions' emotional impact and therapeutic potential.

Professional Boundary Considerations:

Personal therapy should be separate from professional training to maintain appropriate boundaries. Therapists need safe spaces to process their own issues without concern about professional evaluation or training requirements.

Technology and Online Resources

Modern Schema Therapy practice benefits from various technological resources that support learning, practice, and client care.

Online Training Platforms provide access to Schema Therapy education regardless of geographic location. These platforms often include video demonstrations, interactive exercises, and assessment tools.

Clinical Apps and Software support Schema Therapy practice through assessment administration, progress tracking, and homework assignment. Technology can enhance efficiency while maintaining focus on therapeutic relationship and process.

Professional Forums and Discussion Groups provide ongoing consultation and professional development opportunities through online communities of Schema Therapy practitioners.

Ethical Considerations in Schema Therapy Practice

Schema Therapy's intensity and focus on early trauma require careful attention to ethical practice standards. Practitioners must maintain competence, obtain appropriate training, and provide adequate safety for clients engaging in potentially destabilizing work.

Key Ethical Considerations:

Competence Standards require adequate training before practicing Schema Therapy, particularly with complex trauma and personality disorder presentations. Practitioners should work within their competence level and seek supervision when needed.

Informed Consent should include discussion of Schema Therapy's potential emotional intensity, possible temporary destabilization, and requirements for client participation in experiential work.

Safety Planning becomes essential when working with clients who have trauma histories, emotional regulation difficulties, or self-harm behaviors. Practitioners need skills in crisis management and coordination with other providers.

Building Clinical Expertise

Developing Schema Therapy expertise requires systematic skill building across multiple domains: theoretical knowledge, assessment competence, intervention skills, case conceptualization ability, and professional self-awareness.

Skill Development Progression:

Beginning practitioners focus on basic schema assessment and identification while building foundational intervention skills. Intermediate practitioners develop competence in experiential techniques and complex case conceptualization. Advanced practitioners handle severe presentations and provide supervision to others.

Ongoing Learning Opportunities:

Regular case consultation, continuing education, research review, and professional networking support ongoing development throughout a Schema Therapy career. The field's continued growth provides numerous opportunities for learning and contribution.

Specialized Training Areas

Schema Therapy applications continue expanding into specialized areas that require additional training and expertise.

Schema Therapy for Specific Populations:

Training exists for applying Schema Therapy with couples, families, groups, adolescents, and specific diagnostic presentations. Each application requires understanding of population-specific considerations and modified techniques.

Cultural Adaptations:

Schema Therapy training increasingly addresses cultural considerations and adaptations for diverse populations. This includes understanding how schemas might manifest differently across cultures and adapting techniques appropriately.

Contributing to the Field

Experienced Schema Therapy practitioners can contribute to field development through research, writing, training, and clinical innovation. The field benefits from practitioners who share their experiences and develop new applications.

Professional Contribution Opportunities:

Research participation, case study publication, conference presentation, and training assistance provide ways to contribute to Schema Therapy development. These contributions advance the field while supporting individual professional growth.

A Lifetime of Learning

Schema Therapy practice offers rich opportunities for ongoing professional and personal development. The field's continued growth, combined with the complexity and depth of schema work, creates virtually unlimited learning opportunities for committed practitioners.

The investment in Schema Therapy training and development pays dividends not only in improved client outcomes but also in professional satisfaction and growth. Practitioners often find that Schema Therapy enhances their understanding of human psychology and their effectiveness across all therapeutic relationships.

Essential Elements for Professional Development

- ISST training and certification provide structured competence development with quality standards
- Essential literature includes foundational texts, specialized applications, and current research developments
- Ongoing supervision and consultation ensure safe, effective practice while building clinical skills
- Professional organizations offer networking, continuing education, and resource access
- Personal therapy and self-awareness enhance both professional competence and personal growth
- Technology resources support learning, practice efficiency, and professional connection
- Ethical practice requires adequate training, informed consent, and safety planning for intensive emotional work

Appendix F: Safety Guidelines and When to Refer

Schema Therapy's focus on deep emotional processing and early trauma requires careful attention to client safety and appropriate treatment boundaries. While Schema Therapy can be highly effective for complex presentations, certain client characteristics or circumstances may require specialized care, additional support, or alternative treatment approaches[88]. This appendix provides guidance for recognizing when referrals are necessary and maintaining client safety during intensive schema work.

Safety considerations in Schema Therapy extend beyond typical therapy concerns due to the treatment's emphasis on processing childhood trauma, activating vulnerable emotional states, and potentially destabilizing clients before building healthier patterns. Skilled practitioners must balance the benefits of deep emotional work with realistic assessment of client capacity and available support systems.

Assessment of Client Readiness

Not all clients are ready for the intensity of Schema Therapy at the time they present for treatment. Careful assessment helps determine appropriate timing and preparation needed before beginning schema-focused work.

Indicators of Readiness for Schema Work:

Emotional Regulation Capacity sufficient to tolerate moderate emotional distress without becoming overwhelmed or engaging in dangerous behaviors. Clients need baseline ability to self-soothe, tolerate anxiety, and return to equilibrium after emotional activation.

Basic Life Stability including housing, income, and social support adequate to support therapeutic work. Clients dealing with homelessness, severe financial crisis, or complete social isolation may need stabilization before intensive therapy.

Motivation for Deep Work including willingness to examine painful experiences and challenge long-held patterns. Schema Therapy requires active client participation and commitment to difficult emotional work.

Absence of Acute Crisis such as active suicidal ideation, psychotic symptoms, or severe substance abuse that requires immediate intervention before schema work can proceed safely.

Case Example: Premature Schema Work Risks Jennifer, a 28-year-old teacher, sought Schema Therapy for relationship difficulties while dealing with recent job loss, housing instability, and active alcohol abuse. While her relationship schemas were clearly problematic, attempting intensive emotional work during this crisis period would likely increase rather than decrease her distress.

The therapist focused first on crisis stabilization: job search support, temporary housing arrangements, and alcohol treatment referral. Only after Jennifer achieved basic life stability did schema work become appropriate and safe. Rushing into trauma processing during crisis would have been counterproductive and potentially harmful.

Readiness Assessment Guidelines:

- Evaluate current life stressors and crisis factors
- Assess emotional regulation skills and distress tolerance
- Determine availability of social support and professional resources
- Consider client motivation and capacity for sustained therapeutic work
- Identify any acute symptoms requiring immediate intervention

Contraindications for Schema Therapy

Certain presentations require alternative or preparatory treatments before Schema Therapy becomes appropriate. Understanding these contraindications helps prevent harm while ensuring clients receive appropriate care.

Absolute Contraindications:

Active Psychosis including delusions, hallucinations, or severe thought disorder that interferes with reality testing. Clients experiencing psychotic symptoms need psychiatric stabilization before engaging in therapy that might increase confusion or destabilization.

Acute Suicidal Crisis with imminent risk and specific plans requires immediate safety intervention rather than exploratory therapy. Schema work should be postponed until safety is established and maintained.

Severe Cognitive Impairment that prevents understanding of therapeutic concepts or participation in treatment exercises. Clients need sufficient cognitive capacity to engage meaningfully in schema identification and intervention work.

Active Substance Dependence that interferes with memory, emotional regulation, or treatment participation. Addiction treatment should typically precede or occur simultaneously with schema work, with careful coordination between providers.

Relative Contraindications:

Severe Dissociative Disorders may require specialized trauma treatment before schema work becomes safe and effective. Clients with significant dissociation need stabilization and integration work before processing childhood experiences.

Acute Trauma from recent events may need immediate trauma-focused treatment before addressing historical schema patterns. Fresh trauma requires different intervention approaches than developmental schema work.

Severe Personality Disorders with significant behavioral instability may benefit from stabilization-focused treatments like DBT before beginning schema work. Some clients need basic emotional regulation skills before engaging in schema processing.

Case Example: Recognizing Contraindications Michael, a 34-year-old veteran, presented with complex PTSD, active alcohol dependence, and paranoid thoughts about his therapist's motivations. While his trauma history clearly contributed to schema development, his current presentation required different interventions.

The therapist referred Michael for psychiatric evaluation, addiction treatment, and PTSD-specific therapy before considering schema work. Attempting to process childhood trauma while Michael was actively drinking and experiencing paranoid thoughts would have been inappropriate and potentially harmful.

Crisis Management Protocols

Schema Therapy can activate intense emotions and memories that may overwhelm client coping capacity. Having clear crisis management protocols helps maintain safety while supporting continued therapeutic progress.

Crisis Prevention Strategies:

Gradual Exposure to emotional material rather than immediate processing of most traumatic experiences. Building tolerance slowly reduces risk of overwhelming activation.

Between-Session Support including crisis hotlines, emergency contacts, and specific instructions for managing intense emotions outside therapy sessions.

Safety Planning that identifies triggers, early warning signs, and specific steps to take during emotional crises. Plans should include both self-soothing strategies and professional support options.

Medication Coordination with psychiatrists when clients take medications for anxiety, depression, or other conditions that might be affected by intensive emotional work.

Crisis Response Procedures:

When clients become overwhelmed during sessions, therapists should focus on immediate stabilization rather than continuing with planned interventions. This includes grounding techniques, emotional regulation skills, and ensuring client safety before leaving the session.

Between-session crises require clear protocols for contact, assessment, and intervention. Therapists should have emergency contact procedures and clear boundaries about availability and response capabilities.

Case Example: Managing Schema Activation Crisis During an imagery rescripting session, Lisa became overwhelmed with childhood memories and began dissociating. Rather than continuing the imagery work, her therapist focused on grounding techniques and present-moment orientation until Lisa felt stable.

The therapist modified future sessions to include more preparation and safety building before attempting imagery work. This approach prevented repeated overwhelm while maintaining therapeutic progress toward healing goals.

Coordination with Other Providers

Many clients engaged in Schema Therapy benefit from coordination with other mental health providers, medical professionals, or support services. Effective coordination enhances safety while supporting therapeutic goals.

Psychiatric Collaboration:

Clients taking psychiatric medications may need coordination between therapist and psychiatrist, particularly when therapy activates intense emotions that affect medication effectiveness or when medication changes impact therapy participation.

Medical Coordination:

Some clients have medical conditions affected by stress or emotional work. Coordination with primary care providers helps ensure that therapeutic interventions don't adversely affect physical health conditions.

Addiction Treatment Coordination:

Clients with substance abuse histories may need ongoing addiction treatment alongside schema work. Coordination prevents conflicting approaches while addressing both addiction and underlying schema patterns.

Case Example: Integrated Treatment Team Robert, a 41-year-old with bipolar disorder and childhood trauma, worked with a treatment team including a psychiatrist, addiction counselor, and Schema Therapy specialist. Regular communication between providers ensured that therapeutic interventions supported rather than conflicted with each other.

When Robert's mood became unstable during intensive schema work, his psychiatrist adjusted medications while his therapist modified the therapy approach to provide better stabilization. This coordination prevented crisis while maintaining therapeutic progress.

Specialized Referral Situations

Some client presentations require specialized expertise beyond typical Schema Therapy training. Recognizing these situations and making appropriate referrals ensures clients receive optimal care.

Eating Disorders:

While Schema Therapy can be effective for eating disorders, clients with severe medical complications or acute risk require specialized eating disorder treatment with medical monitoring and nutritional rehabilitation.

Severe Trauma and Dissociation:

Clients with extensive trauma histories and dissociative symptoms may benefit from trauma specialists who have additional training in complex PTSD and dissociative disorders before or alongside schema work.

Personality Disorders with Severe Behavioral Instability:

Some clients with borderline or other personality disorders need intensive stabilization treatment before schema work becomes appropriate. DBT or residential treatment may be necessary precursors to schema therapy.

Couples and Family Issues:

When schema patterns significantly affect family functioning, clients may benefit from family therapy or couples work in addition to individual schema therapy. Some situations require systemic intervention alongside individual work.

Documentation and Legal Considerations

Schema Therapy's intensity requires careful documentation and attention to legal and ethical considerations that protect both clients and therapists.

Documentation Requirements:

Thorough assessment documentation including contraindication screening, readiness evaluation, and safety planning. Progress notes should reflect ongoing safety assessment and any crisis interventions used.

Informed Consent:

Clients should understand Schema Therapy's potential emotional intensity, possible temporary destabilization, and requirements for active participation in potentially difficult exercises. Consent should address crisis procedures and therapist availability.

Risk Assessment:

Regular evaluation of suicide risk, self-harm potential, and other safety concerns. Documentation should reflect ongoing risk assessment and any safety interventions implemented.

Legal Consultation:

Complex cases may benefit from legal consultation about documentation requirements, duty to warn obligations, and other legal considerations relevant to intensive emotional therapy.

Training and Competence Requirements

Therapists providing Schema Therapy should have adequate training and ongoing supervision, particularly when working with complex trauma and personality disorder presentations.

Minimum Training Standards:

Basic Schema Therapy training through recognized programs, with additional specialized training for complex presentations. Therapists should work within their competence level and seek consultation when needed.

Ongoing Supervision:

Regular supervision or consultation, particularly during skill development phases and when working with high-risk clients. Complex cases benefit from ongoing professional support and guidance.

Personal Therapy:

Therapists benefit from understanding their own schema patterns and how these might affect their work with clients. Personal therapy isn't required but is strongly recommended for professional and personal development.

Building a Safety Culture

Effective Schema Therapy practice requires a culture of safety that prioritizes client wellbeing while supporting therapeutic progress. This includes realistic assessment of treatment readiness, appropriate preparation for intensive work, and willingness to modify approaches based on client response.

Safety culture also involves recognizing the limits of individual therapist competence and making appropriate referrals when specialized expertise is needed. The goal is ensuring that clients receive optimal care rather than trying to provide all services within a single therapeutic relationship.

Protection Through Preparation

The best safety approach in Schema Therapy involves thorough preparation rather than crisis response. Careful assessment, gradual exposure, adequate support systems, and realistic treatment planning prevent most safety concerns while supporting effective therapeutic outcomes.

When safety concerns do arise, prompt recognition and appropriate response minimize harm while often providing opportunities for therapeutic growth and learning. Crisis situations, when handled skillfully, can strengthen rather than damage the therapeutic relationship and process.

References

1. Young, J. E., Klosko, J. S., & Weishaar, M. E. (2003). *Schema therapy: A practitioner's guide*. New York: Guilford Press.
2. Arntz, A., & Jacob, G. (2013). *Schema therapy in practice: An introductory guide to the schema mode approach*. John Wiley & Sons.
3. Young, J. E., & Klosko, J. S. (1993). *Reinventing your life: The breakthrough program to end negative behavior and feel great again*. New York: Dutton.
4. Rafaeli, E., Bernstein, D. P., & Young, J. (2011). *Schema therapy: Distinctive features*. New York: Routledge.
5. Jacob, G. A., & Arntz, A. (2013). Schema therapy for personality disorders—A review. *International Journal of Cognitive Therapy*, 6(2), 171–185.
6. Young, J. E., Klosko, J. S., & Weishaar, M. E. (2007). *Schema therapy: A practitioner's guide* (Revised edition). New York: Guilford Press.
7. Farrell, J. M., Shaw, I. A., & Webber, M. A. (2009). A schema-focused approach to group psychotherapy for outpatients with borderline personality disorder: A randomized controlled trial. *Journal of Behavior Therapy and Experimental Psychiatry*, 40(2), 317-328.
8. Yalcin, O., Lee, C. W., & Correia, H. (2020). Factor structure of the Young Schema Questionnaire (Long Form-3). *Australian Psychologist*, 55(5), 546-558.
9. Young, J. E. (2005). *Young Schema Questionnaire–Short Form 3* (YSQ-S3). New York: Schema Therapy Institute.
10. Welburn, K., Coristine, M., Dagg, P., Pontefract, A., & Jordan, S. (2002). The schema questionnaire—short form: Factor analysis and relationship between schemas and symptoms. *Cognitive Therapy and Research*, 26(4), 519-530.
11. Maslow, A. H. (1943). A theory of human motivation. *Psychological Review*, 50(4), 370-396.
12. Young, J. E., Klosko, J. S., & Weishaar, M. E. (2003). *Schema therapy: A practitioner's guide*. New York: Guilford Press.

13. Arntz, A., & Jacob, G. (2013). *Schema therapy in practice: An introductory guide to the schema mode approach*. John Wiley & Sons.
14. Edwards, D. J. (2003). The schema therapy model. In J. Beck, A. Freeman, D. Davis, & Associates (Eds.), *Cognitive therapy of personality disorders* (pp. 45-67). New York: Guilford Press.
15. Farrell, J. M., Shaw, I. A., & Webber, M. A. (2009). A schema-focused approach to group psychotherapy for outpatients with borderline personality disorder: A randomized controlled trial. *Journal of Behavior Therapy and Experimental Psychiatry*, 40(2), 317-328.
16. Bamelis, L. L., Evers, S. M., Spinhoven, P., & Arntz, A. (2014). Results of a multicenter randomized controlled trial of the clinical effectiveness of schema therapy for personality disorders. *American Journal of Psychiatry*, 171(3), 305-322.
17. Arntz, A., & Weertman, A. (1999). Treatment of childhood memories: Theory and practice. *Behaviour Research and Therapy*, 37(8), 715-740.
18. Smucker, M. R., & Niederee, J. (1995). Treating incest-related PTSD and pathogenic schemas through imaginal exposure and rescripting. *Cognitive and Behavioral Practice*, 2(1), 63-93.
19. Kellogg, S. (2004). *Dialogical encounters: Contemporary perspectives on chairwork in psychotherapy*. Psychotherapy: Theory, Research, Practice, Training, 41(3), 310-320.
20. Paivio, S. C., & Greenberg, L. S. (1995). Resolving "unfinished business": Efficacy of experiential therapy using empty-chair dialogue. *Journal of Consulting and Clinical Psychology*, 63(3), 419-425.
21. Beck, A. T., Freeman, A., & Associates. (1990). *Cognitive therapy of personality disorders*. New York: Guilford Press.
22. Young, J. E., Klosko, J. S., & Weishaar, M. E. (2003). *Schema therapy: A practitioner's guide*. New York: Guilford Press.
23. Beck, J. S. (2011). *Cognitive behavior therapy: Basics and beyond* (2nd ed.). New York: Guilford Press.
24. Young, J. E., Klosko, J. S., & Weishaar, M. E. (2003). *Schema therapy: A practitioner's guide*. New York: Guilford Press.
25. Leahy, R. L. (2003). *Cognitive therapy techniques: A practitioner's guide*. New York: Guilford Press.

26. McManus, F., Van Doorn, K., & Yiend, J. (2012). Examining the effects of thought records and behavioral experiments in instigating belief change. *Journal of Behavior Therapy and Experimental Psychiatry*, 43(1), 540-547.
27. Padesky, C. A. (1994). Schema change processes in cognitive therapy. *Clinical Psychology & Psychotherapy*, 1(5), 267-278.
28. Rafaeli, E., Bernstein, D. P., & Young, J. (2011). *Schema therapy: Distinctive features*. New York: Routledge.
29. Smucker, M. R., & Niederee, J. (1995). Treating incest-related PTSD and pathogenic schemas through imaginal exposure and rescripting. *Cognitive and Behavioral Practice*, 2(1), 63-93.
30. Arntz, A., & Weertman, A. (1999). Treatment of childhood memories: Theory and practice. *Behaviour Research and Therapy*, 37(8), 715-740.
31. Kellogg, S. (2004). *Dialogical encounters: Contemporary perspectives on chairwork in psychotherapy*. Psychotherapy: Theory, Research, Practice, Training, 41(3), 310-320.
32. Paivio, S. C., & Greenberg, L. S. (1995). Resolving "unfinished business": Efficacy of experiential therapy using empty-chair dialogue. *Journal of Consulting and Clinical Psychology*, 63(3), 419-425.
33. Welburn, K., Coristine, M., Dagg, P., Pontefract, A., & Jordan, S. (2002). The schema questionnaire—short form: Factor analysis and relationship between schemas and symptoms. *Cognitive Therapy and Research*, 26(4), 519-530.
34. Maslow, A. H. (1943). A theory of human motivation. *Psychological Review*, 50(4), 370-396.
35. Young, J. E. (2005). *Young Schema Questionnaire–Short Form 3* (YSQ-S3). New York: Schema Therapy Institute.
36. Yalcin, O., Lee, C. W., & Correia, H. (2020). Factor structure of the Young Schema Questionnaire (Long Form-3). *Australian Psychologist*, 55(5), 546-558.
37. Edwards, D. J. (2003). The schema therapy model. In J. Beck, A. Freeman, D. Davis, & Associates (Eds.), *Cognitive therapy of personality disorders* (pp. 45-67). New York: Guilford Press.
38. Farrell, J. M., Shaw, I. A., & Webber, M. A. (2009). A schema-focused approach to group psychotherapy for outpatients with borderline personality disorder: A

randomized controlled trial. *Journal of Behavior Therapy and Experimental Psychiatry*, 40(2), 317-328.

39. Bamelis, L. L., Evers, S. M., Spinhoven, P., & Arntz, A. (2014). Results of a multicenter randomized controlled trial of the clinical effectiveness of schema therapy for personality disorders. *American Journal of Psychiatry*, 171(3), 305-322.

40. Linehan, M. M. (2014). *DBT Skills Training Manual* (2nd ed.). New York: Guilford Press.

41. Deci, E. L., & Ryan, R. M. (2000). The "what" and "why" of goal pursuits: Human needs and the self-determination of behavior. *Psychological Inquiry*, 11(4), 227-268.

42. Siegel, R. D. (2009). *The mindfulness solution: Everyday practices for everyday problems*. New York: Guilford Press.

43. Kabat-Zinn, J. (2003). *Mindfulness-based interventions in context: Past, present, and future. Clinical Psychology: Science and Practice*, 10(2), 144-156.

44. Neff, K. (2011). *Self-compassion: The proven power of being kind to yourself*. New York: William Morrow.

45. Van der Kolk, B. A. (2014). *The body keeps the score: Brain, mind, and body in the healing of trauma*. New York: Penguin Books.

46. Johnson, S. M. (2019). *Attachment in psychotherapy*. New York: Guilford Press.

47. Hazan, C., & Shaver, P. (1987). Romantic love conceptualized as an attachment process. *Journal of Personality and Social Psychology*, 52(3), 511-524.

48. Van der Kolk, B. A. (2014). *The body keeps the score: Brain, mind, and body in the healing of trauma*. New York: Penguin Books.

49. Yalom, I. D., & Leszcz, M. (2020). *The theory and practice of group psychotherapy* (6th ed.). New York: Basic Books.

50. Farrell, J. M., Shaw, I. A., & Webber, M. A. (2009). A schema-focused approach to group psychotherapy for outpatients with borderline personality disorder: A randomized controlled trial. *Journal of Behavior Therapy and Experimental Psychiatry*, 40(2), 317-328.

51. Lambert, M. J. (2013). *Outcome in psychotherapy: The past and important advances. Psychotherapy*, 50(1), 42-51.

52. Kraus, D. R., Seligman, D., & Jordan, J. R. (2005). Validation of a behavioral health treatment outcome and assessment tool designed for naturalistic settings: The treatment outcome package. *Journal of Clinical Psychology*, 61(3), 285-314.
53. Young, J. E., Klosko, J. S., & Weishaar, M. E. (2003). *Schema therapy: A practitioner's guide*. New York: Guilford Press.
54. Diener, E., Emmons, R. A., Larsen, R. J., & Griffin, S. (1985). The satisfaction with life scale. *Journal of Personality Assessment*, 49(1), 71-75.
55. Beck, A. T., Steer, R. A., & Brown, G. K. (1996). *Manual for the Beck Depression Inventory-II*. San Antonio, TX: Psychological Corporation.
56. Norcross, J. C., & Prochaska, J. O. (2002). Using the stages of change. *Harvard Mental Health Letter*, 18(11), 5-7.
57. Young, J. E., Klosko, J. S., & Weishaar, M. E. (2003). *Schema therapy: A practitioner's guide*. New York: Guilford Press.
58. Linehan, M. M. (2014). *DBT Skills Training Manual* (2nd ed.). New York: Guilford Press.
59. Neff, K. (2011). *Self-compassion: The proven power of being kind to yourself*. New York: William Morrow.
60. Lambert, M. J. (2013). *Outcome in psychotherapy: The past and important advances*. *Psychotherapy*, 50(1), 42-51.
61. Rafaeli, E., Bernstein, D. P., & Young, J. (2011). *Schema therapy: Distinctive features*. New York: Routledge.
62. Beck, A. T., Freeman, A., & Associates. (1990). *Cognitive therapy of personality disorders*. New York: Guilford Press.
63. Johnson, S. M. (2019). *Attachment in psychotherapy*. New York: Guilford Press.
64. Van der Kolk, B. A. (2014). *The body keeps the score: Brain, mind, and body in the healing of trauma*. New York: Penguin Books.
65. Kabat-Zinn, J. (2003). *Mindfulness-based interventions in context: Past, present, and future*. *Clinical Psychology: Science and Practice*, 10(2), 144-156.
66. Siegel, R. D. (2009). *The mindfulness solution: Everyday practices for everyday problems*. New York: Guilford Press.
67. Deci, E. L., & Ryan, R. M. (2000). The "what" and "why" of goal pursuits: Human needs and the self-determination of behavior. *Psychological Inquiry*, 11(4), 227-268.

68. Hazan, C., & Shaver, P. (1987). Romantic love conceptualized as an attachment process. *Journal of Personality and Social Psychology*, 52(3), 511-524.
69. Yalom, I. D., & Leszcz, M. (2020). *The theory and practice of group psychotherapy* (6th ed.). New York: Basic Books.
70. Farrell, J. M., Shaw, I. A., & Webber, M. A. (2009). A schema-focused approach to group psychotherapy for outpatients with borderline personality disorder: A randomized controlled trial. *Journal of Behavior Therapy and Experimental Psychiatry*, 40(2), 317-328.
71. Kraus, D. R., Seligman, D., & Jordan, J. R. (2005). Validation of a behavioral health treatment outcome and assessment tool designed for naturalistic settings: The treatment outcome package. *Journal of Clinical Psychology*, 61(3), 285-314.
72. Diener, E., Emmons, R. A., Larsen, R. J., & Griffin, S. (1985). The satisfaction with life scale. *Journal of Personality Assessment*, 49(1), 71-75.
73. Beck, A. T., Steer, R. A., & Brown, G. K. (1996). *Manual for the Beck Depression Inventory-II*. San Antonio, TX: Psychological Corporation.
74. Leahy, R. L. (2003). *Cognitive therapy techniques: A practitioner's guide*. New York: Guilford Press.
75. McManus, F., Van Doorn, K., & Yiend, J. (2012). Examining the effects of thought records and behavioral experiments in instigating belief change. *Journal of Behavior Therapy and Experimental Psychiatry*, 43(1), 540-547.
76. Padesky, C. A. (1994). Schema change processes in cognitive therapy. *Clinical Psychology & Psychotherapy*, 1(5), 267-278.
77. Smucker, M. R., & Niederee, J. (1995). Treating incest-related PTSD and pathogenic schemas through imaginal exposure and rescripting. *Cognitive and Behavioral Practice*, 2(1), 63-93.
78. Arntz, A., & Weertman, A. (1999). Treatment of childhood memories: Theory and practice. *Behaviour Research and Therapy*, 37(8), 715-740.
79. Kellogg, S. (2004). *Dialogical encounters: Contemporary perspectives on chairwork in psychotherapy*. Psychotherapy: Theory, Research, Practice, Training, 41(3), 310-320.
80. Paivio, S. C., & Greenberg, L. S. (1995). Resolving "unfinished business": Efficacy of experiential therapy using

empty-chair dialogue. *Journal of Consulting and Clinical Psychology*, 63(3), 419-425.

81. Welburn, K., Coristine, M., Dagg, P., Pontefract, A., & Jordan, S. (2002). The schema questionnaire—short form: Factor analysis and relationship between schemas and symptoms. *Cognitive Therapy and Research*, 26(4), 519-530.

82. Maslow, A. H. (1943). A theory of human motivation. *Psychological Review*, 50(4), 370-396.

83. Young, J. E., Klosko, J. S., & Weishaar, M. E. (2003). *Schema therapy: A practitioner's guide*. New York: Guilford Press.

84. Arntz, A., & Jacob, G. (2013). *Schema therapy in practice: An introductory guide to the schema mode approach*. John Wiley & Sons.

85. Bamelis, L. L., Evers, S. M., Spinhoven, P., & Arntz, A. (2014). Results of a multicenter randomized controlled trial of the clinical effectiveness of schema therapy for personality disorders. *American Journal of Psychiatry*, 171(3), 305-322.

86. Rafaeli, E., Bernstein, D. P., & Young, J. (2011). *Schema therapy: Distinctive features*. New York: Routledge.

87. International Society of Schema Therapy. (2023). *Training and certification standards*. Retrieved from https://www.schematherapysociety.org

88. Young, J. E., Klosko, J. S., & Weishaar, M. E. (2003). *Schema therapy: A practitioner's guide*. New York: Guilford Press.

89. Farrell, J. M., & Shaw, I. A. (2018). *Experiencing schema therapy from the inside out: A self-practice/self-reflection workbook for therapists*. New York: Guilford Press.

90. Loose, C., Graaf, P., & Zarbock, G. (2013). *Störungsspezifische Schematherapie mit Kindern und Jugendlichen* [Disorder-specific schema therapy with children and adolescents]. Weinheim: Beltz.

91. Sempértegui, G. A., Karreman, A., Arntz, A., & Bekker, M. H. (2013). Schema therapy for borderline personality disorder: A comprehensive review of its empirical foundations, effectiveness and implementation possibilities. *Clinical Psychology Review*, 33(3), 426-447.

92. Roediger, E., Stevens, B. A., & Brockman, R. (2018). *Contextual schema therapy: An integrative approach to*

personality disorders, emotional dysregulation, and interpersonal functioning. Oakland, CA: Context Press.

www.ingramcontent.com/pod-product-compliance
Lightning Source LLC
Chambersburg PA
CBHW070737270326
41927CB00010B/2020